HUMAN SEXUALITY
Second Edition

Kenneth L. Jones
Louis W. Shainberg
Curtis O. Byer
Mt. San Antonio College

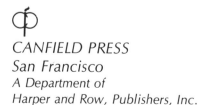
CANFIELD PRESS
San Francisco
A Department of
Harper and Row, Publishers, Inc.

HUMAN SEXUALITY, Second Edition

Copyright © 1975 by Kenneth L. Jones, Louis W. Shainberg, and Curtis O. Byer

Library of Congress Cataloging in Publication Data

Jones, Kenneth Lamar, 1931-
    Human sexuality.

    First ed. published in 1970 under title: Marriage
and reproduction.
    Bibliography
    Includes index.
    1. Sex. 2. Marriage. I. Shainberg, Louis W.,
joint author. II. Byer, Curtis O., joint author.
III. Title. [DNLM: 1. Marriage. 2. Reproduction.
HQ734 J77m]
HQ31.J67 1975   612.6   75-2486
ISBN 0-06-384321-8

Interior and cover design by Penny Faron

PREFACE

Eldon E. Quine

This book, one of a series by the same authors on various topics in health science, discusses the biological, psychological, sociological, and ethical aspects of human sexuality. We wrote the book to fill several needs. One is to provide the information and attitudes an individual needs to decide how to best express his own sexuality. Another is to help the individual avoid such specific problems as unwanted pregnancy, unhappy marriage, and sexual dysfunction. Still another is to help the reader achieve a sense of sexual adequacy, an important part of a positive self-concept.

We have selected the topics in this book on the basis of our experience in college courses in health science and human sexuality and years of open communication with young people, both inside and outside the college classroom.

Sexuality is discussed in various contexts—marital, nonmarital, extramarital, and homosexual relationships. Special emphasis is placed on the interaction of sexuality and society, especially in areas of controversy.

K.L.J.
L.W.S.
C.O.B.

CONTENTS

Chapter 1
SEX AND SOCIETY

We sometimes talk of society as if it were a mysterious entity all its own, but in truth a society is simply a group of individuals. This fact is the basis of social conflict about sex. The sexual attitudes held by individuals cover a wide and contradictory range; what seems right and good to one may be evil to another. And, to make matters worse, there is no simple solution to such conflict. The issues of male and female sex roles, sexual freedom, sexual ethics, nonmarital sexual adjustment, marriage and its alternatives, and the presentation of sex in the arts and media are exceptionally complex.

At the social level, the continual conflict between sexual suppression and sexual freedom is evidenced by controversy and courtroom battles. At the same time, each person undergoes an internal conflict, attempting to reconcile personal desires and needs with moral upbringing, parental standards, and social pressures. Recent, more enlightened social attitudes toward sexuality certainly contribute to greater personal satisfaction and individual freedom, but they also complicate the problem, eliminating hard-and-fast standards of sexual conduct and allowing a greater latitude that may itself embroil the person in internal conflict.

Sex and Personality

In the early days of psychiatry, primarily because of the work of Sigmund Freud, it was customary to attribute all kinds of psychological problems to sexual causes. Today, however, prevalent professional opinion has reversed itself, holding that most sexual problems have a psychological cause. Of course, it's obvious that many emotional problems have little or no sexual element and that some sexual problems have nothing to do with the mind. However, psychiatry is quite right in assigning sexuality a major role in personality.

The sex drive is one of the basic human drives and thus has both obvious and hidden effects on personality. Our degree of sexual satisfaction influences how we respond to people of both sexes. Sexual satisfaction is usually associated with a more relaxed personality, with increased tolerance for frustrations of all kinds. Sexual dissatisfaction has been related to irritability, aggression, inability to tolerate frustration, and mild neuroses.

A central theme throughout this book is the development of a sense of sexual adequacy, an important part of one's self-concept. A secure feeling of sexual adequacy is very much a part of a healthy sense of self-esteem. How one perceives one's own sexual adequacy strongly influences his or her behavior. Someone who feels inadequate often sets out to "prove" sexual adequacy, both through exaggerated sexual activity and through intensive participation in activities stereotypical of his or her sex. Someone who feels very inadequate may go to the extreme of avoiding direct sexual relationships entirely, though the individual may still engage in many nonsexual activities that confirm his or her sexual role. By contrast, a secure sexuality allows honest, relaxed, and satisfying sexual and nonsexual relationships.

Sex Roles

The most significant sexual controversy in American society today concerns male and female roles—the expectations and limitations that society imposes on each sex. Many people are strongly dissatisfied with sex-role stereotypes. Others resist any change in the status quo just as emphatically, perhaps because redefinition of sex roles would challenge their own sense of masculinity or femininity.

An important question today is how greatly sex roles are determined by purely cultural factors as opposed to inborn physical or mental differences between the sexes. There is no clear answer to this question.

In every known society certain duties were performed predominantly by women, certain tasks reserved for men, and certain jobs left without sexual assignment. However, the specific jobs assigned to each sex varies from society to society. A task seen as masculine in one society may be feminine in another. There are, however, certain consistencies among the majority of societies. For example, men are more typically assigned tasks that are physically strenuous or that involve long periods away from home. Female activities are more often less strenuous, more solitary, and more closely tied to the home. From a biological viewpoint, some authorities have speculated that this arrangement evolved because of the greater physical strength of the male and the need for the mother to stay near her nursing baby.

Keep in mind that this arrangement is not necessarily valid for a technological society such as ours. Very few jobs really require more physical strength than the majority of women possess. Many professions in which physical strength is no factor at all are essentially closed to women.

Sexual prejudice against females is still very much a reality in the United States. Sadly, even many women have been conditioned to believe that they are inferior and should be subordinate to men. Despite the efforts of women's groups and the fair employment practice laws, women in the United States have, in the past 40 years, actually lost ground in both professional status and educational attainment as compared to men. In 1930, half of the professional and semiprofessional workers were women, but today only about a third are. In the 1930s, about one in every seven Ph.D. degrees was awarded to a woman, while today the ratio is closer to one in ten. Most major religions of the United States (and the world) relegate women to a second-class status, reserving the more important positions for men. In every phase of their lives—occupational, political, religious, and social—women encounter a tremendous reservoir of sexual prejudice from both men *and* other women.

It is obvious that rigidly spelled-out sex roles artificially limit the possibilities for self-fulfillment. Anyone whose interests and abilities happen to belong to areas the culture has assigned to the opposite sex is saddled with frustration.

While strict sex role delineation can be unjustly limiting, many authorities feel that a complete lack of any sex role development would also detract from mental health and adjustment. Clearly, our society would most benefit from a balanced, open view of each person's capabilities.

One of the ways a society influences the sexual attitudes, behavior, and roles of its members is through *modeling,* the process in which an individual observes and adopts as his own the attitudes and behavior of other people. Parents are the primary models for sexual roles, but there are many others. The image of women in the media, for example, is particularly influential. While it could be argued that the media merely reflect the real place of women in our society, a strong case can be made that women are often portrayed in a degrading way and that this portrayal definitely influences how men perceive the role of women and how women view themselves.

The liberation of both sexes requires considerable individual self-confidence. The self-confidence of many of today's women is good evidence that they have finally seen themselves as competent, self-determining individuals. A woman should realize that being meek and dependent is not necessarily attractive. Success and femininity are not incompatible; no woman is obliged to put up with sexist references to her and her abilities. Now, if men could only develop enough self-confidence, especially in regard to their masculinity, they would see that a woman can be "liberated" and still be feminine—an interesting companion, a professional colleague, a good sex partner and, if she so desires, a competent wife and mother. The self-confident male would not see such a woman as a threat to his masculinity.

Sexual Behavior and Society

Every society has shown a concern about the sexual behavior of its members typically expressed as a set of sexual "do's and dont's," some of which are maintained as cultural customs and expectations, while others are enforced as laws. The standards for sexual behavior in a society typically evolve from several sources. A primary concern in most societies, and certainly in our own, is the welfare of the child. Since the child depends on adults for many years, many laws and customs exist to ensure a secure and stable home for the child. The traditional restriction of sexual intercourse to marriage is an example of an attempt to ensure that a child is born into a stable relationship where adequate child care is assured.

But many of society's other sexual conventions have little or nothing to do with child security and have evolved to protect the individual from exploitation, to prevent behavior that is offensive to certain other individuals, or to reflect various religious dogmas. Many laws fall into this category, such as those concerning homosexuality, nudity, pornography, oral and anal sex, and prostitution. Laws such as these, which try to regulate morality, are currently being challenged as creating "crimes without victims." Many people argue that any form of private sexual behavior between mutually consenting adults in which no one is harmed ought to be legal.

Conflicting standards of sexual behavior present a greater problem in the United States than in many other countries, possibly because of the great diversity of cultural and religious backgrounds in the population. There can be little doubt that these conflicts and controversies will be with us for some time to come.

Changing Attitudes

The traditional attitude of Western culture toward sexual expression has been one of repression and prohibition, based on the puritan ethic of work, self-denial, and duty. That which is done to produce or accomplish something material or permanent is good, especially if it isn't much fun. On the other hand, play, self-indulgence, purposelessness, and spontaneity are bad and dangerous. Such attitudes have been reinforced by the church, the state, and even medicine and psychiatry, which should have known better. Sex was seen as solely for the purpose of reproduction and possibly for the expression of "marital love," with the kind of sexual expression sharply limited. All other sexual behaviors were classified as "perversions," crimes, sins, or, worst of all, as illnesses. Masturbation, oral and anal sex, nonmarital sexual intercourse, and homosexual love all met with varying degrees of disapproval. Male and female social roles were also strictly defined.

But in the past 15 or 20 years, there have been many obvious and subtle changes. The central trend of these changes has been to free sexual thought and action from the traditional restraints. The so-called sexual revolution really consists of an increasingly widespread recognition that a mindless conformity to moral strictures on acceptable sexual activity, whether imposed by state, church, or family, is neither necessary nor desirable for the individual or for society. Ultimately, the sexual revolution is an expression of individual demands for sexual self-determination, a dawning of the awareness that the nature of one's sexual activity can and should be a matter of conscious personal choice based on one's own needs and desires, coupled with a genuine concern for the rights and needs of others.

Knowledge is the foundation of all valid and useful decisions. Few areas of personal experience are as important as the development of healthy, satisfying sexual attitudes, and yet few areas get so little solid and compassionate attention. This book serves to right that balance.

Defining Some Terms

The terminology used in this book to distinguish various sexual contexts is slightly unconventional.

To describe relations outside marriage in which the partners have no direct plans to marry, we generally prefer "nonmarital" to "premarital." Nonmarital is less restrictive than premarital, including not only the unmarried but also the divorced and widowed. "Marital" relations are those between spouses during marriage. "Extramarital" are those relations carried on by either spouse in an ongoing marriage with someone outside the marriage.

Summary

I. Sex and Personality

A. Psychological problems once customarily attributed to sexual causes

B. Today opposite is true—sexual problems seen as having psychological causes

C. Sex drive has obvious and subtle influences on personality

D. A central theme of this book is development of sense of sexual adequacy

II. Sex Roles

A. Much controversy today on male and female roles

B. An important question is the extent to which sex roles are culturally (vs. inherently) determined. No answer yet

C. Male and female roles vary among different societies

D. Society influences sexual roles through modeling

E. Liberation of both sexes from stereotyped roles will require individual self-confidence—insecure person senses a threat to sense of masculinity or femininity

III. Sexual Behavior and Society

A. Conflicting standards of sexual behavior a great problem in the United States

B. Controversy likely to continue for many years

IV. Changing Attitudes

A. Traditional attitude of Western culture toward sexual expression has been repressive

B. Many changes in sexual attitudes and behavior in recent years

C. "Sexual revolution" has been a recognition of the need for sexual self-determination

V. Defining Some Terms

A. Nonmarital—refers to relations outside marriage when partners have no direct plans to marry

B. Marital—between spouses during marriage

C. Extramarital—relations carried on by either spouse with someone outside the marriage while marriage is in effect

Questions for Review

1. List some ways in which sex roles are stereotyped in our culture. Do any of these role-assignments seem to be based on basic, or inherent, differences between females and males? Explain.

2. What is meant by modeling of sex roles?

3. How does the sense of sexual adequacy relate to our liberation from stereotyped sex roles?

4. What is meant by sexual self-determination?

Chapter 2
SEXUAL ANATOMY AND PHYSIOLOGY

A thorough knowledge of the biological aspects of both sexes is important to an understanding of human sexuality. Familiarity with sexual anatomy and physiology contributes to an appreciation of the mechanisms of normal sexual response, an understanding of the common problems in sexual response, the effective use of many forms of birth control, and the health of both mother and child in pregnancy.

The Male Reproductive Organs

We will consider the male organs in the sequence that a sperm encounters them from formation to ejaculation from the body.

The Testes and the Production of Sperm

The primary reproductive organs (gonads) of the male are a pair of testes, also called testicles. Each testis is an oval gland about 1½ inches long. The testes are suspended from the under side of the body in a bag, the scrotum (Figures 2.1 and 2.2). Sperm production cannot occur at normal body temperatures. The scrotum allows the testes to be suspended from the

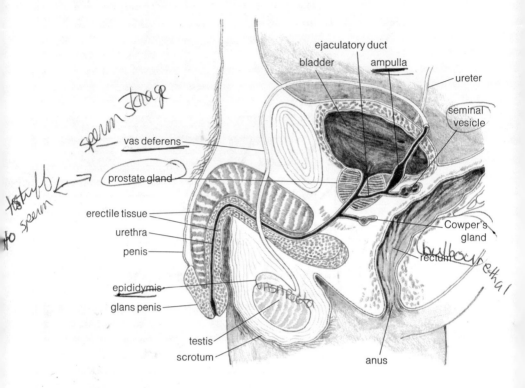

Figure 2.1   *Male reproductive system (side view)*

body, where their temperature is three to four degrees lower than normal body temperature. In cold temperatures, the thin scrotal muscles contract and pull the testes closer to the body wall; in hot temperatures, the muscles relax, allowing the testes to be dropped farther away. The scrotum is supplied with abundant sweat glands, which also contribute to cooling in hot temperatures.

In the developing male fetus, the testes originate in the abdominal cavity. By the eighth month of pregnancy, the testes descend from the abdominal cavity to the scrotum.

The testes produce hormones as well as sperm. Hormones are chemical messengers produced in one part of the body and carried by the blood to regulate the functions and development of other parts. The production of male sex hormones increases sharply with the onset of puberty, marking the beginning of the physical changes leading to sexual maturity. Such changes are called *secondary sex characteristics* and include the development of broad shoulders, lowered voice, growth of hair on the face, chest, and pubis, and development of the male sex drive.

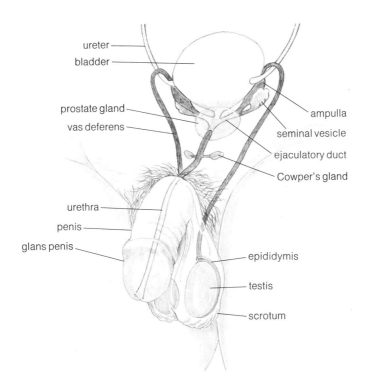

Figure 2.2 *Male reproductive system (front view)*

Each testis contains a great number of very small tubes called *seminiferous tubules* (Figure 2.3), where the sperm cells are formed. Beginning at puberty, these sperm cells are produced more or less continuously throughout life. Initial production starts slowly, then increases, until, in the sexually mature male, the incredible number of ten to thirty billion sperm is produced each month. The number of sperm produced during a man's lifetime defies imagination.

Each sperm cell is microscopic in size. One sperm is about 50 microns long; it would take 480 of them placed end to end to cover an inch. The sperm consists of a head, neck, body, and tail (Figure 2.4). One set of chromosomes (23 in number) is carried in the head. These chromosomes bear the male's contribution to the heredity of his offspring.

Epididymis

As the sperm develop, they move out of the seminiferous tubules and collect in a coiled tube called the *epididymis*. It lies on the upper side of

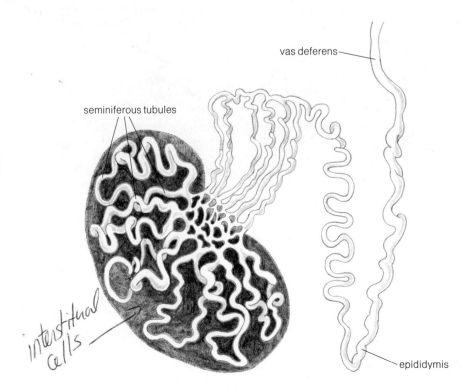

Figure 2.3   *Structure of human testis*

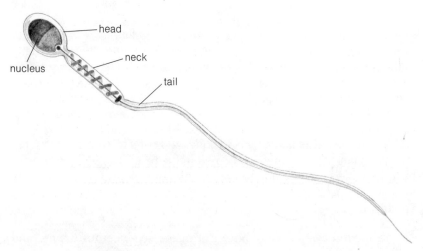

Figure 2.4   *Human sperm cell*

each testis and would be about 20 feet long if uncoiled. Here sperm mature and are stored until released from the body by ejaculation or until they disintegrate and are reabsorbed.

Vas Deferens

The *vas deferens* is a duct about 18 inches long that carries sperm from the epididymis to the *ejaculatory duct* (Figure 2.1). Near the ejaculatory duct is an enlarged section called the *ampulla* which, like the epididymis and vas deferens, stores sperm. During ejaculation, the walls of the vas deferens contract, propelling sperm cells through the duct.

Seminal Vesicles

The *seminal vesicles* are a pair of glands located at the base of the urinary bladder in front of the rectum (Figure 2.1). They empty into the vas deferens to form the ejaculatory duct. During ejaculation, the vesicles contract and add their clear, sticky, glandular secretions to the semen.

Prostate Gland

This large organ is located directly below the bladder (Figure 2.1). It surrounds the *urethra* (duct carrying urine from the bladder to the end of the penis). The ejaculatory ducts pass through each side of the prostate gland to join the urethra. During ejaculation the gland contracts to add its milky secretions to the semen.

In older men, the prostate gland commonly enlarges so that it obstructs the urethra, thus hindering urination. This condition occurs to some degree in over half of all elderly men and can usually be corrected surgically.

Bulbourethral (Cowper's) Glands

Two small glands about the size of peas lie on either side of the urethra slightly below the prostate gland (Figure 2.1). These glands produce a mucus secretion that precedes ejaculation and appears at the tip of the penis as a drop of clear, sticky liquid. This secretion serves to remove any urine in the present urethra and to help lubricate the vaginal canal in intercourse.

Penis

The male organ of sexual intercourse is the *penis* (Figures 2.1 and 2.2). Containing the urethra, this organ is used both for urine excretion and for the ejaculation of semen. As with other organs, the size of the penis varies. An average erect penis is about six inches in length and one inch in diameter. Passing through the length of the penis are three columns of erectile tissue, two *corpora cavernosa* and a smaller *corpus spongiosum*, seen in the cross section of the penis in Figure 2.5. At the tip of the penis, the corpus

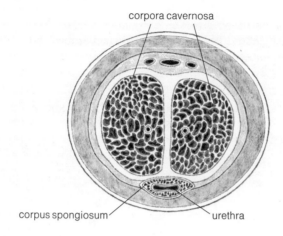

corpora cavernosa

corpus spongiosum   urethra

Figure 2.5   *Cross section of the penis showing erectile tissues*

spongiosum enlarges to form the *glans penis*. The glans penis's rich supply of nerve receptors makes it especially sensitive to external stimulation. A free fold of skin called the *foreskin*, or *prepuce*, overhangs the glans penis when it is relaxed. To prevent infection of the glans penis, the foreskin is often removed surgically in the operation known as *circumcision*.

Semen

Semen, or *seminal fluid*, is the gray-white, sticky liquid ejaculated during the male orgasm. It consists of sperm cells from the testes plus secretions from the seminal vesicles, prostate gland, and bulbourethral glands. Both the volume of semen ejaculated and the number of sperm it contains vary. The volume depends on the frequency of ejaculation, while the sperm content is influenced by frequency of ejaculation and the rate of sperm production. Frequent or repeated ejaculation temporarily reduces both the volume and sperm content of the ejaculate.

Male Reproductive Hormones

The male sex hormones are collectively called _androgens_. A principal androgen, called *testosterone*, is produced by the testes. It is formed by cells between the seminiferous tubules called _interstitial cells_. Testosterone is responsible for the development of male secondary sexual characteristics as well as for development of the reproductive organs.

Occasionally, a deficiency of gonadotropic (gonad-stimulating) hormones from the pituitary gland or other conditions cause the testes to produce too little testosterone. The removal of the testes, called *castration*, may also cause hormonal deficiencies in the male. Since the production of testosterone becomes increasingly important to the male after the time of puberty, the effects of insufficient testosterone depend on the timing of the deficiency. If it happens before puberty, the male fails to develop male secondary sex characteristics. A boy who loses his testes prior to puberty is known as a eunuch. If a male loses the testes after the onset of puberty, he will retain some male secondary sex characteristics and lose others. Injectable and oral forms of testosterone are available to treat testosterone deficiency.

The Female Reproductive Organs

The internal female organs include the ovaries, Fallopian tubes, uterus, and vagina. The external organs consist of the hymen, labia majora and minora, and clitoris.

Ovaries

Eggs (ova) are produced in the *ovaries* (female gonads). They are situated deep in the pelvic cavity, one on either side of the uterus (Figures 2.6 and 2.7). Each is attached to the uterus by a ligament.

The ovaries serve a dual function, producing both eggs and hormones.

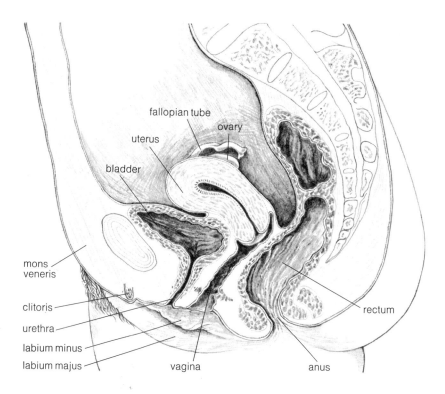

Figure 2.6 *Female reproductive system (side view)*

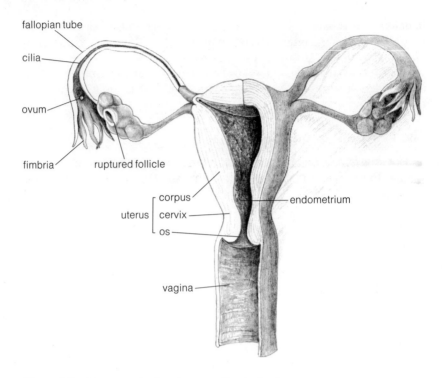

fallopian tube

cilia

ovum

fimbria

ruptured follicle

corpus

uterus   cervix

os

endometrium

vagina

Figure 2.7   *Uterus and related organs (front view)*

Within the ovary are many *ovarian follicles*. At the time of birth, the ovaries contain an estimated 400,000 immature follicles, each housing an immature egg. Beginning with puberty, these immature follicles ripen or mature at the rate of one about every 28 days and develop into *Graafian follicles*. Each month, usually midway between menstrual discharges, a Graafian follicle ruptures and releases a mature egg. Since the reproductive life of the female extends about 35 years (ages 12 to 47) and about one egg per 28 days is produced (or 13 per year), only about 375 eggs out of a possible 400,000 ever mature.

Each Graafian follicle begins development near the center of the ovary. As it enlarges, it moves outward until it finally appears like a little blister on the surface of the ovary (Figure 2.8). Near the midpoint between menstrual discharges, it ruptures and releases the egg within it, a process called *ovulation*. After ovulation, a blood clot forms at the place of the ruptured follicle. The blood clot is soon replaced by yellow-colored cells and is called a *corpus luteum,* which remains about 12 days.

Fallopian Tubes

The *Fallopian tubes,* or *oviducts,* are some 4 inches long and extend from the uterus out to the ovaries. Fertilization usually occurs in the Fallopian tubes. The outer end of each tube is fringed *(fimbriated),* and

mature graafian follicle   developing follicles

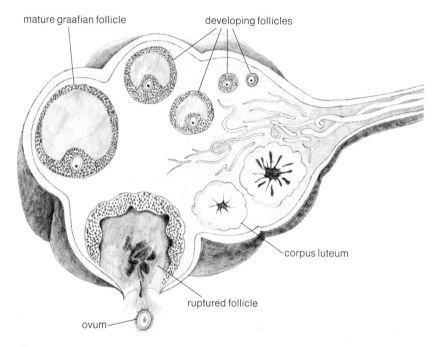

corpus luteum

ruptured follicle

ovum

Figure 2.8 *Cross section of ovary showing ovarian follicles*

these fingerlike fringes *(fimbria)* are adjacent to each ovary (Figure 2.7). The fimbria catch the egg and pass it into the Fallopian tube. The inner lining of the tube is covered with minute, hairlike structures called *cilia*. Once inside the Fallopian tube, the egg is propelled toward the uterus by movements of the cilia and by contractions in the walls of the tube. The egg cannot move on its own.

Once the egg is released from the ovary, it can be fertilized by any sperm which may be present. An egg is believed to remain viable for about 24 hours, after which it begins to degenerate; fertilization must take place within about 24 hours after ovulation if conception is to occur that month.

Uterus

The *uterus* (womb) is a hollow, pear-shaped organ located in the pelvis (Figure 2.6). It is slightly above and behind the bladder, but in front of the rectum, and loosely suspended by several ligaments. Normally the uterus tilts forward. Loosening of the ligaments due to childbearing may tilt the uterus backward. Other causes for displacement can be pelvic disease (such as cancer) and congenital deformity. The uterus is typically about 3 inches long and 2 inches wide in the adult. Its walls are thick and very muscular. In pregnancy it stretches to over 12 inches in length to accommodate the growing baby. The upper half of the uterus is the *corpus* (body), the lower half the *cervix*, and the lower opening is the *os*.

The inner lining of the uterus, the *endometrium*, is richly supplied with blood vessels and glands. Following ovulation, the egg descends through the tube into the uterus, a journey requiring three to four days. If it has been fertilized, it becomes embedded in the endometrium within four to five days after entering the uterus (or seven to eight days after fertilization).

Vagina

The *vagina* is a tube extending from the external genitalia to the uterus (Figure 2.6). This muscular tube is 4 to 6 inches long, and lies between the bladder and the rectum. It serves as the excretory duct for the uterus, as the female organ for intercourse, and as the birth canal in childbirth. Sexual arousal causes glands in the vaginal lining to secrete a lubricant that eases intercourse.

Hymen

In young girls, the external opening of the vagina may be partially closed by a membrane called the *hymen*. This membrane varies in size and thickness, and may remain intact until first intercourse. It may, however, be greatly reduced in size from the use of tampons (a vaginal insert used during menstrual discharge), from a physician's manipulation during a medical examination, or from participation in active sports. In a few cases the hymen may need to be surgically cut or stretched by a physician before intercourse can be accomplished. Contrary to common belief, rupture of the hymen may not involve bleeding.

The Labia

Two pairs of liplike structures surround the external opening of the vagina (Figure 2.9). The outer and larger pair are the *labia majora*; the inner and smaller pair are the *labia minora*. The space between the labia minora, into which the vaginal passageway and the urethra open, is the *vestibule*.

Clitoris

Directly in front of the vestibule is a small erectile organ called the *clitoris* (Figure 2.9). During sexual arousal it becomes erect through engorgement with blood, and is the chief site of sexual excitement in the female. Unlike the penis, the clitoris does not contain the urethra.

The fatty cushion on the surface of the body directly in front of the labia majora is the *mons veneris*. During the time of puberty, it becomes covered with pubic hair.

The Menstrual Cycle

Menstruation is the periodic discharge of blood, mucus, and cellular fragments from the uterine lining (see Figure 2.7), occurring at more or less

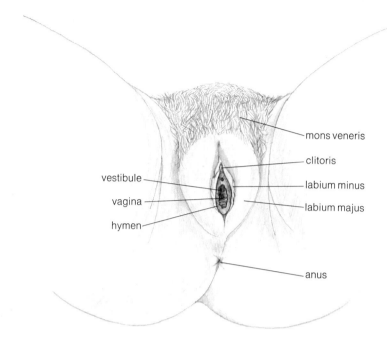

Figure 2.9 *Female external genital organs*

regular intervals (except during pregnancy and lactation) from the time of puberty to the menopause.

Menstruation commonly begins between the twelfth and thirteenth year, but may start as early as the tenth year or as late as the sixteenth. First menstruation is referred to as *menarche*. Since puberty is the broad range of physical changes that occurs between childhood and maturity, menarche represents just one aspect of puberty.

The cessation of menstruation, or *menopause*, commonly occurs near 47 years of age. About half of all women cease menstruating between 45 and 50 years of age, about a quarter before 45, and about a quarter after 50. As the menarche represents just one sign of puberty, so menopause is just one sign of the *climacteric*, sometimes called the "change of life."

Although menstrual discharge most commonly occurs every 28 days, women vary considerably in the length of their *menstrual cycles*, or the interval of days between discharges. Some women have cycles as short as 18 days and others as long as several months. In fact, with many women, the length of the menstrual cycle varies from cycle to cycle.

The menstrual flow usually lasts three to five days, but periods ranging from two to eight days may be considered normal for some women. For a given woman, the duration of the flow is commonly the same month after month.

Certain contraceptive methods influence menstruation. Women taking oral contraceptives, for example, typically experience shorter, lighter periods, while women with intrauterine devices (IUDs) often have heavier than average periods.

Usually the discharge is liquid, although clots may appear if the flow is excessive. The average amount of blood lost ranges from 25 to 60 milliliters (about 2 to 4 tablespoons) each menstruation.

Some women report a weight gain of one to three pounds just before the beginning of menstrual discharge. This is retained water rather than fat.

The cycle of events in the uterus from the beginning of one menstrual discharge until the next is called the *menstrual cycle*. Four phases can be observed during the typical 28-day cycle: (1) the proliferative or follicular phase, (2) the ovulatory phase, (3) the secretory or luteal phase, and (4) the destructive or menstrual phase (Figure 2.10). The first day of the menstrual discharge is referred to as Day 1.

Proliferative or Follicular Phase

After menstruation has stopped (Days 3–5 of the cycle), the uterine lining is thin (Figure 2.10). The glands in the lining are straight, short, and narrow. In

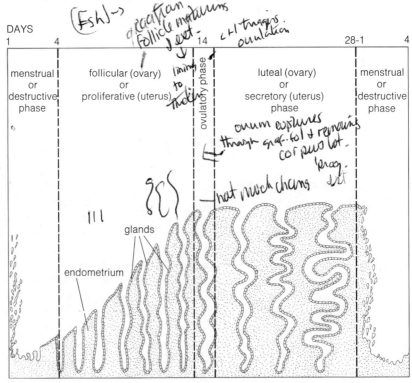

Figure 2.10 *Diagram showing cyclic changes in thickness of endometrium and endometrial glands during menstrual cycle*

the ovary, the Graafian follicle is maturing. During this phase, which lasts about 10 days, the follicle produces a hormone, *estrogen*, that causes the uterine lining to become thick and dense.

Ovulatory Phase

Ovulation usually occcurs between Days 12 and 16, but may fall earlier or later in the cycle. During the day of ovulation there is little change in the uterine lining. As soon as the ovum ruptures through the Graafian follicle, the remains of the follicle become a corpus luteum.

Secretory or Luteal Phase

progesterone

Under the influence of hormones given off by the corpus luteum, the uterine lining continues to thicken. The glands in the lining become enlarged, twisted, and very active. This phase of the cycle lasts 13 to 14 days. In the event the egg is not fertilized, the corpus luteum folds in and becomes inactive. The production of luteal hormones falls off, and the cells and glands of the lining begin to die, causing the destructive phase, or menstrual flow. If the egg is fertilized, it becomes embedded in the uterine lining where it continues to develop.

Destructive or Menstrual Phase

This phase occurs because of the death of the cells in the uterine lining. This layer has a very rich blood supply. Disintegration of the lining causes a sloughing of blood and cell remains. This phase usually lasts three to five days, and is evident as the menstrual flow.

Hormones and the Menstrual Cycle

The menstrual cycle is under the control of two sets of hormones, those from the anterior pituitary gland, called gonadotropic hormones, and those from the ovary.

Gonadotropic Hormones

The *pituitary gland* is located at the base of the brain (Figure 2.11). Its *anterior* (front) portion produces three hormones that regulate the female gonads (ovaries) and are called the *gonadotropic hormones*. The name and effect of each is as follows.

Hormone	Effect
Follicle-stimulating hormone (FSH)	FSH directs the development and activity of the Graafian follicles. It causes the follicles to secrete estrogen.

Hormone	Effect
Luteinizing hormone (LH)	LH works with FSH to stimulate continued estrogen production. It triggers ovulation, thereby initiating formation of the corpus luteum and causing it to begin secreting both estrogen and progesterone.
Luteotropic hormone (LTH)	LTH is responsible for increased secretion of estrogen and progesterone by the corpus luteum. It increases in production as LH decreases. It causes milk secretion by the mammary glands after the birth of the baby.

Ovarian Hormones

Under the stimulation of the gonadotropic hormones, the ovaries secrete two hormones, *estrogen* and *progesterone*.

ESTROGEN

Estrogen is produced by the Graafian follicle before ovulation and by the corpus luteum after ovulation. It brings about the maturation of the secon-

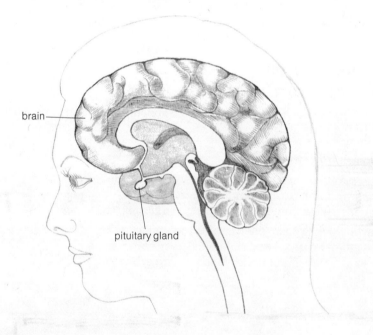

Figure 2.11   *Location of pituitary gland at base of brain*

dary female characteristics, including development of the breasts, deposition of fat around the hips, growth of hair in the pubic area, maturation of the reproductive tract, and initiation of the female sexual drive. Complete removal of the ovaries (oophorectomy) before puberty prevents the development of secondary sex characteristics, and the sexual organs remain immature. Removal after puberty causes the cessation of menstruation, and the body becomes more masculine. Estrogen also stimulates the growth of the uterine lining during the proliferative phase of the cycle.

Increased amounts of estrogen feed back to the pituitary gland, causing it to slow down FSH production and to speed up LH production. As seen in Figure 2.12, this occurs during the proliferative phase.

PROGESTERONE

Progesterone is produced by the corpus luteum. It prepares the uterine lining for the implantation of a fertilized egg. In pregnancy, progesterone maintains the lining in good condition. During pregnancy, it is produced by the corpus luteum during the first two to three months and by the placenta (see page 91) thereafter for the course of the pregnancy.

If there is no pregnancy, increased amounts of progesterone in the blood feed back to the pituitary gland, slowing LH production and thus causing the corpus luteum to dry up.

Oral contraceptives prevent pregnancy by affecting this feedback response. The synthetic estrogen and/or progesterone in the pills inhibits the production of gonadotropic hormones, thus preventing the maturation of the eggs and ovulation.

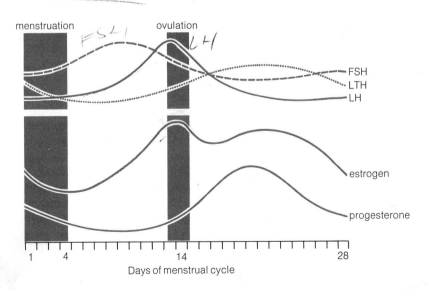

Figure 2.12 *Hormone levels during typical menstrual cycle*

Summary

I. The Male Reproductive Organs

    A. The testes and the production of sperm

        1. Male gonads are pair of testes (testicles)

        2. Scrotum keeps testes at temperature lower than body's

        3. Testes produce hormones as well as sperm

    B. Epididymis—coiled tube in which sperm mature

    C. Vas deferens

        1. Duct carrying sperm up into abdomen

        2. Upper end (ampulla) stores mature sperm

    D. Seminal vesicles—contribute fluid to semen

    E. Prostate gland—also produces seminal fluid

    F. Bulbourethral (Cowper's) glands—pair of small glands producing preejaculatory fluid

    G. Penis

        1. Contains urethra, carrying both semen and urine

        2. Contains spongy erectile tissues

    H. Semen—mixture of sperm and fluid released during male orgasm

    I. Male reproductive hormones

        1. Collectively called androgens

        2. Principal androgen is testosterone, produced by testes

II. The Female Reproductive Organs

    A. Ovaries—the female gonads

        1. Produce ova (eggs) and hormones

        2. Each contains thousands of immature follicles, each containing an immature egg

    B. Fallopian tubes (oviducts)

        1. Carry egg from ovary to uterus

        2. Lined with cilia

        3. Usual site of fertilization

    C. Uterus (womb)

        1. Contains fetus in pregnancy

        2. Cervix (neck) extends into vagina

D. Vagina

    1. Organ of intercourse and birth canal

    2. Lining secretes lubricant during sexual arousal

E. Hymen

    1. A membrane that may partially cover opening of vagina

    2. Variable in extent

F. Labia—two pairs of liplike structures surrounding opening of vagina

    1. Labia majora—outer pair

    2. Labia minora—inner pair

G. Clitoris

    1. Small erectile organ above opening of vagina

    2. Site of sexual pleasure

III. The Menstrual Cycle

  A. Menstruation—the periodic discharge of products of breakdown of uterine lining

  B. Menarche—onset of first menstrual period

  C. Menopause—cessation of menstrual cycles

  D. Phases:

    1. Proliferative or follicular—egg is maturing, uterine lining is building up

    2. Ovulatory phase—egg ruptures from follicle, empty follicle converts to corpus luteum

    3. Secretory or luteal phase—uterine lining ready to receive fertilized egg, corpus luteum secreting progesterone

    4. Destructive or menstrual phase—uterine lining breaking down (menstrual period)

IV. Hormones and the Menstrual Cycle   *→ regulate female ovaries*

  A. Gonadotropic hormones—from pituitary gland

    1. Follicle-stimulating hormone (FSH)—stimulates maturity of follicle and egg and promotes secretion of estrogen

    2. Luteinizing hormone (LH)—stimulates ovulation, formation of corpus luteum, and secretion of estrogen and progesterone

    3. Luteotropic hormone (LTH)—increases secretion of estrogen and progesterone

  B. Ovarian hormones—secreted by ovaries

    1. Estrogen—produced by Graafian follicle and corpus luteum *estrogen*

a. Stimulates development of secondary sex characteristics

b. Stimulates growth of uterine lining

c. Inhibits production of FSH and stimulates production of LH by pituitary

2. Progesterone—produced by corpus luteum

a. Prepares uterine lining for fertilized egg

b. Maintains uterine lining (prevents menstruation)

c. Inhibits production of LH by pituitary

3. Action of oral contraceptives based on inhibition of gonadotropic hormones

Questions for Review

1. Trace the path of a sperm cell from its origin to its ejaculation from the body.

2. What are the sources of seminal fluid? *seminal veside, prostrate glanc bou/barethad*

3. Why are the male and female gonads considered dual-purpose organs?

4. What are androgens? *male sex hormones*

5. Where is the egg usually fertilized?

6. What is the source of the menstrual discharge?

7. What are the phases of the menstrual cycle?

8. What are gonadotropic hormones?
   gonad stimulating

gonad- primary reproductive organ

Chapter 3
SEXUAL RESPONSE

Only in recent years has human sexual response become a respectable field for scientific research. Prior to that time, there was little objective investigation. Some people felt that sex was dirty or sacred or that its mystery was best preserved in the absence of study. Scientists who could have been studying sex were themselves inhibited by their own insecurity or prudishness. Finally, since sexual inadequacy is not a major cause of death, the research funds available for studies on cancer or heart disease were not to be had by sex researchers.

Sex research on a large scale was first popularized in the late 1940s and the 1950s by the Kinsey group, who interviewed large numbers of persons about their sex histories and habits. This study caused a major uproar. Society doesn't accept data about sex at face value the way it does data in other areas of biological and medical research. Rather, each portion of society, each religion, and each social class imposes its own values on this material. Some people saw the Kinsey research as a passport from the darkness to the light, while to others it was the work of some insidious and evil conspiracy. The problem remains. When Masters and Johnson published their excellent works on sexual response and inadequacy in 1966 and 1970, they met with much the same response that Kinsey had met twenty years earlier.

Objective sex research is of obvious value. It places sexuality in its proper perspective as a normal part of human physiology and behavior. It removes the cloak of secrecy from sexuality. It dispels anxiety by showing people that their sexual activity and desires are indeed typical. And, for those with true sexual problems, it provides the kind of solid information needed to build good therapy.

Sexual Stimuli

Sexual responses are a basic element of human physiology and psychology. Not surprisingly, they can be induced by a wide range of stimuli—the sounds, smells, touch, sight; and indeed even the thought of sexual situations can sexually arouse most people.The sexual response of both male and female can be divided into identifiable phases, each with its physical and emotional characteristics.

The *excitement phase* is the first, accompanied by the initial signs of physical arousal. The *plateau phase* follows, in which the sex organs further change in size and shape. Breathing and cardiac rates increase. The *orgasm phase* brings the intensely satisfying sensations of sexual climax. In the *resolution phase*, the organs return to their normal sizes and shapes, and the intense feelings of climax subside.

Sexual Response in the Male

The excitement phase in the male is signaled by erection of the penis. The erectile tissue is a spongy mass of blood-filled spaces. During sexual arousal, the small arteries supplying blood to the penis dilate, letting more blood in, while the small veins draining the erectile tissue contract, letting less blood out. Thus blood accumulates in the penis, producing erection—an increase in width, length, and firmness. The scrotum tightens, and the testes draw up close to the body (Figure 3.1).

Erection may be brought on by physical contact with the penis, sexual thoughts, sights or sounds, or by involuntary activity of the nervous system during sleep. When sexual arousal is prolonged, the penis may erect and relax and then erect again several times.

In the plateau phase, the fully erect penis may increase in diameter as orgasm approaches, particularly around the glans, and may turn a reddish-purple color. A few drops of preejaculatory fluid from the Cowper's glands are gradually emitted from the penis. The testes become further elevated (the more complete the testicular elevation, the greater the ejaculatory pressure), and they increase in size. A sex flush (reddening of the skin) may appear, rate of breathing and heart rate increase, and muscular tension develops over various body parts.

The increase in sexual arousal to the point of orgasm (ejaculation) requires, in all but a very few males, tactile stimulation of the penis, though in a highly aroused man orgasm may follow a very brief contact. Masters and Johnson divide the male orgasm into two stages. The first stage is a period of two or three seconds before ejaculation during which the male can feel the ejaculation coming and can in no way restrain or control it. The second stage is the actual ejaculation of semen from the penis by contractions of the urethra and related muscles. The first three or four contractions expel the semen under great pressure. During orgasm, the breathing rate may increase to over 40 times per minute, and the heart rate to from 110 to 180 or more beats per minute.

Involuntary ejaculation occurring during sleep is called a *nocturnal emission* ("wet dream"). This is accompanied by an orgasm and is a perfectly normal and harmless event.

In the resolution phase, following ejaculation, the penis usually reduces quickly to about half its erect dimensions, then more slowly to its unstimulated size. During the few minutes immediately after ejaculation, the glans of the penis may be painfully sensitive to touch. The scrotal sac gradually reverts to its relaxed state, and the testes descend.

The majority of men are incapable of another erection for an hour or more after ejaculation. However, the minimum time interval required before repeated male erection and orgasm varies greatly, both among different men and for the same man at different times. It may range from minutes to days. This time interval increases with the age of the man and with general physical or emotional fatigue, but it is decreased by the degree of original sexual arousal, the degree of sexual restimulation after ejaculation, and the period of sexual restraint prior to the first ejaculation. If the man is young, has been without sexual release for some time, or is restimulated after ejaculation, he may be ready for further sexual intercourse within just a few minutes.

Female Sexual Response

The response of a woman's body to sexual stimulation is widespread, involving organs besides the genitalia. In the excitement phase, the clitoris increases two or three times in size; the labia majora and labia minora expand and spread. The vagina may begin to lubricate within ten to twenty seconds, the outer two-thirds lengthening and distending. The uterus moves away from the vagina. Lubrication varies among females, yet for a given woman it usually depends on how aroused she is. During excitement, the breast enlarges, and the nipple erects, stiffens, becomes highly sensitive to touch, and flushes. The areola (the dark ring around the nipple) is engorged with blood (Figure 3.2). Skeletal muscles contract throughout the body. Pulse and breathing rates increase.

At the plateau phase, the clitoris moves under its hood and becomes so tender that efforts to touch it directly may produce discomfort. The labia minora increase in size and turn bright red. The outer one-third of the vagina contracts, while the inner two-thirds expands.

In the orgasm phase, strong contractions occur in the outer half of the vagina (three to five in a mild orgasm, eight to twelve in an intense one). The uterus contracts as it does in labor, and the anus contracts tightly. The intensity and duration of orgasm in the female varies more than in the male.

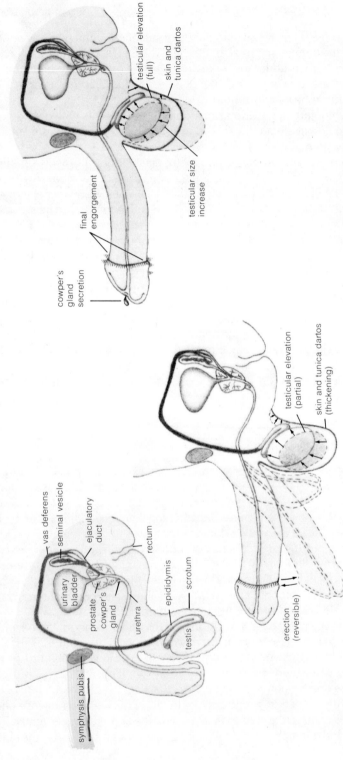

A. Male pelvic organs during the unexcited or normal phase.

symphysis pubis

vas deferens
seminal vesicle
ejaculatory duct
urinary bladder
rectum
prostate
cowper's gland
urethra
epididymis
scrotum
testis

B. Male pelvic organs during the excitement phase.

testicular elevation (partial)
skin and tunica dartos (thickening)
erection (reversible)

C. Male pelvic organs during the plateau phase.

testicular elevation (full)
skin and tunica dartos
testicular size increase
final engorgement
cowper's gland secretion

Figure 3.1 *Stages in male sexual arousal*

D. *Male pelvic organs during the orgasmic phase.*

E. *Male pelvic organs during the resolution phase.*

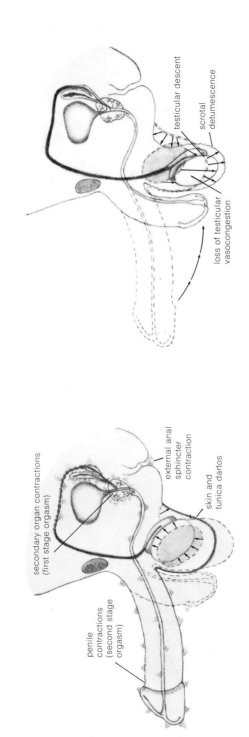

secondary organ contractions (first stage orgasm)

penile contractions (second stage orgasm)

external anal sphincter contraction

skin and tunica dartos

testicular descent

scrotal detumescence

loss of testicular vasocongestion

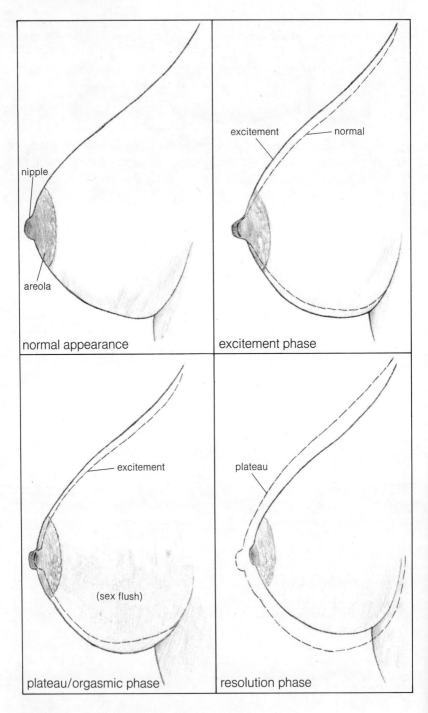

Figure 3.2   *Breast response to sexual stimulation*

In the resolution phase, the clitoris and labia slowly return to normal size and position. The outer one-third of the vagina quickly returns to normal, while the inner two-thirds returns to normal more slowly (five to eight minutes). Following orgasm, the sex flush of the breasts rapidly disappears, and the breast size slowly (five to ten minutes) returns to normal.

The period of sexual stimulation preceding orgasm varies from woman to woman and from time to time for the same woman. The experience of many couples is that the woman needs a longer period of stimulation in intercourse to achieve orgasm than does the man. But Kinsey et al. (1953) reported that the average woman can masturbate to orgasm almost as fast as the average man. They attributed the difference to the fact that the masturbating woman can manipulate her sensitive areas more specifically than is possible in intercourse. This conclusion seems to be confirmed by Masters and Johnson (1966), who found the measurable physiologic intensity of female orgasm greatest in masturbation, moderate in partner manipulation, and lowest in intercourse.

The subjective experiences of a woman during orgasm, as reported by Masters and Johnson, begin with a feeling that orgasm is imminent, followed by an intense sensual awareness of the pelvic region. The woman becomes almost completely oblivious to the surrounding environment, focusing on her own sensations. The next feeling, reported by almost every woman, is that of warmth, starting in the pelvic region and spreading throughout the body. A final feeling, reported consistently, is that of a pelvic throbbing.

During and directly following orgasm there is a marked coolness of the lips of the mouth and surrounding areas. This is due to sudden release of blood vessels. Muscular and psychological relaxation accompanies orgasm.

Caressing of the clitoris plays an important role in achieving orgasm for many women, yet clitoral stimulation is not essential in achieving orgasm. A sexually responsive woman whose clitoris is removed surgically will remain capable of orgasm in intercourse. Some women can achieve orgasm when a part of the body distant from the clitoris, such as the ear canal or the small of the back or the anus, is stimulated. Even where the clitoris is not stimulated directly, it enlarges and participates fully in the total response. A woman's body responds to stimulation consistently regardless of the source of that stimulation. There is neither a purely clitoral orgasm nor a purely vaginal one, but from the body's point of view only one kind, a sexual orgasm.

Many women are multi-orgasmic (experiencing three or more orgasms within a few minutes) if stimulation is repeatedly resumed before sexual arousal drops below plateau-phase levels. Masturbation often best contributes to multi-orgasmic ability, because it frees the woman from dependence on her partner's abilities. In intercourse, the possibilities for multiple orgasm depend somewhat on the partner's ejaculatory control—

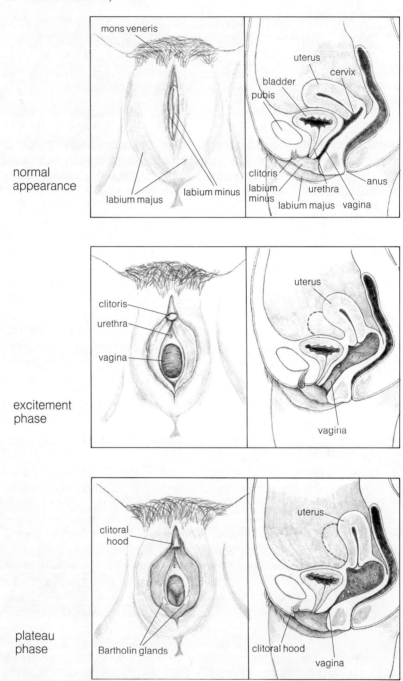

Figure 3.3   *Response of female genitalia (external and internal) to sexual stimulus*

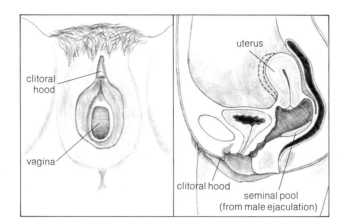

orgasmic
phase

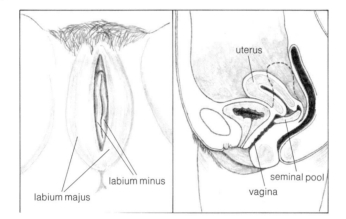

resolution
phase

Figure 3.3 *(Cont.)*

his ability to engage in prolonged, vigorous intercourse without ejaculation and subsequent loss of erection. Many women also enjoy reaching multiple orgasms through oral or manual stimulation by their partners.

The Nervous System and Sexual Response

Sexual responses are controlled by the autonomic (involuntary) nervous system. While this portion of the nervous system is not under direct conscious control, it does respond strongly to a person's emotional state.

The autonomic nervous system is split into two subdivisions (see Table 3.1). One of these, the *parasympathetic* branch, is activated by a sense of well-being to restore and conserve energy. This branch is responsible for sexual arousal.

The other subdivision of the autonomic nervous system, the *sympathetic* branch, is activated by such emotions as fear, worry, anxiety, anger, and hostility to prepare the body for emergency action. This branch inhibits sexual arousal, and excessive action of the sympathetic branch can completely block sexual response. Since emotional disturbance or distress can stimulate the sympathetic branch almost constantly, it is not surprising that many emotional problems have sexual side effects.

Sexual Techniques

The authors are not going to give detailed instruction or step-by-step formulas for achieving sexual satisfaction, because we believe that attempts to follow such instructions can actually hinder, rather than help, a couple in attaining this goal. We feel that a good sexual relationship can be achieved if each partner has adequate knowledge of sexual psychology and physiology, a positive attitude toward sex, and a concern for the sexual satisfaction of the partner. Open and uninhibited discussion of sexual desires and responses is more important than the "rules" in some book. Each partner should feel free to tell the other which practices increase sexual enjoyment and which decrease it. An interest in sexual experimentation is good, especially after several years of marriage; but no couple satisfied with their sexual relationship should feel a need to experiment simply because experiment has suddenly become chic. Partners should act as their own guides rather than relying on some authority outside the relationship.

Before Intercourse

There is no set routine universally necessary or useful in preparing for intercourse. The sexual responses of individual men and women are highly variable and individual, so a technique ideal for one couple may have no value for another.

It is common, however, for the woman to need more stimulation before intercourse than the man, in order to prevent pain upon first penetration and increase her chances of achieving orgasm. While a man may attain erection in a few seconds, a woman may need several minutes to become fully aroused and produce adequate vaginal lubrication.

Most people enjoy a few minutes of sexual foreplay to prepare them physically and psychologically for successful, pleasurable intercourse. Most women, for example, discover particular types of caresses and stimuli which provide them with the most intense sensations, and they should freely communicate this information to their partners. Among the types of sex play that stimulate many women are kissing; kissing the ears and neck; gently fondling or tightly squeezing the breasts; lightly rubbing, pinching, pulling, sucking, or lip-biting the nipples; squeezing or lightly rubbing the buttocks; lightly stroking the insides of the thighs; and oral and hand manipulation of the genital organs. Genital manipulation is mentioned last because many women prefer to become somewhat aroused before this begins. Many books recommend direct manipulation of the clitoris, but Masters and Johnson (1966) suggest that since direct stimulation of the clitoris can be painful, most women prefer indirect stimulation through manipulation of the mons veneris.

Men similarly respond to a great variety of stimuli, such as kissing; licking and kissing the ears; body kisses; and oral and manual stimulation of the nipples, penis, scrotum and testes, and anus. In sex play, any practice accepted and enjoyed by both partners has its place.

In all types and phases of sexual relationships, open and honest communication is important. Many people are very reluctant to talk about sex, even to the extent that they fail to tell their partners just what pleases or displeases them sexually. Therapists report many cases where the primary cause of sexual problems is lack of communication between partners. It is of utmost importance that couples develop the ability to openly and honestly communicate their sexual feelings.

Sexual Intercourse

The different positions used successfully for sexual intercourse are frankly innumerable. Many sex manuals have stressed positions that bring the penis into direct contact with the clitoris, working from the assumption that the greatest amount of stimulation of the most sensitive part of the female body must be best. However, the research of Masters and Johnson (1966) and the personal experience of many couples indicate that such contact actually decreases the sexual pleasure of both the man and the woman. Sexual positions in which the clitoris receives indirect stimulation are more satisfactory for the majority of women and probably all men. Any position that allows the penis to fully penetrate the vagina will provide an adequate amount of indirect clitoral stimulation.

A couple who try many different positions for intercourse will probably find several that seem particularly good for them and will probably use all of these positions from time to time. There are many variations for the basic positions discussed below.

MAN-ABOVE POSITIONS

These are probably the most common positions in use in the United States and they seem to be the most natural and comfortable positions for many couples. The woman lies on her back with her legs spread apart, either drawn up or straight out. The man lies facing her, between her thighs. This position allows most couples to kiss freely but restricts breast manipulation more than some of the other positions.

WOMAN-ABOVE POSITIONS

In these common positions, the man lies on his back while the woman lies or sits above and facing him. Some couples roll from the man-above to the woman-above or vice versa. Some women can achieve orgasm more easily in the woman-above position by controlling the pelvic thrusts, while the man is more or less passive.

FACE-TO-FACE SIDE POSITIONS

These positions offer several advantages. Neither partner must support the weight of the other, so they are good for prolonged sexual connections. Kissing is easy, as is breast manipulation or any other type of caress desired.

REAR-ENTRY POSITIONS

There are several different basic rear-entry positions. The woman may lie on her side or face down or may kneel on her hands and knees. In any case, the man approaches from behind, passing his erect penis between her legs and into her vagina.

OTHER POSITIONS

The variety of sexual positions is limited only by the imagination and agility of the couple. Many couples occasionally use a more unusual position to add variety to their love-making. The sitting positions are one such variation. In one sitting position, the man may sit on a chair or the edge of a bed while the woman sits astride him. Some couples enjoy intercourse while standing up, using front or rear entry. There is no reason why any position that affords mutual pleasure should not be used.

After the penis has been fully inserted into the vagina, a man is often at the very peak of his sexual arousal and near orgasm. In order to prevent premature ejaculation, many couples find it desirable to lie together quietly for a short time before beginning the pelvic thrusts of intercourse. By lying quietly at this time and any subsequent time that orgasm seems near, many men can delay ejaculation for some time without loss of erection.

The pelvic thrusts may be made by the man or the woman or both together. Many couples use all three types of movements. The speed and depth of the thrusts can be increased to intensify sexual arousal or decreased to delay orgasms and prolong the connection. Most couples must pace their movements carefully to bring the woman to orgasm without causing premature orgasm in the male. Breast and nipple stimulation increase the level of arousal of most women and many men. Many people respond intensively to kissing of their ears, necks, and shoulders. Some couples find that a pillow placed under the hips of the woman helps intensify the sensation of the penis within the vagina.

Factors Affecting Orgasm

It is important to keep in mind, however, that the best evidence suggests that position is not the crucial variable in coital orgasm. Masters and

Johnson have named fatigue and preoccupation as the two major deterrents.

Attainment of orgasm seems to be more closely related to length of foreplay. Gebhard found that, with foreplay of 21 or more minutes, only 8 percent of women had no orgasm. The duration of intercourse was also related to orgasm. Virtually no woman had coital orgasm with less than one minute of intercourse, while 95 percent of women reached orgasm after intercourse of 16 or more minutes.

No single pattern of orgasm is best for every couple, though many couples find, through experimentation, a pattern that seems best for them. Many couples develop a pattern whereby the woman reaches one or more orgasms first, followed by the ejaculation of the man. In other couples, the woman finds that the stimulus of the penis throbbing in ejaculation is just what she needs to reach orgasm.

The degree of satisfaction resulting from orgasm varies among individuals and even from orgasm to orgasm for the same individual. Often, even though there is full physiological orgasm, little pleasurable sensation is associated with it, and little or no emotional satisfaction. This evidence of the strong psychological element in sexual response shows why true sexual satisfaction usually depends more on a good relationship between the partners than on sexual gymnastics.

Frequency of Intercourse

The frequency of sexual intercourse is a source of conflict in many relationships. In almost any relationship, there will be times when one partner would like sexual intercourse and the other partner is either not interested or is incapable of responding. Such situations may place a great burden upon the relationship unless both partners are understanding and tolerant. Some sex manuals have portrayed the ideal relationship as a continuous sexual spree with each orgasm bigger and better than the one previous. In reality, sex is only a part of the total man-woman relationship, and the success of a couple's sexual relationship is often a reflection of their total interaction.

Various research projects have indicated that the average man would like to engage in intercourse a little more often than would his partner. Of course, in a particular couple there may be a great similarity in sexual desire or very great differences, with either partner having the greater desire.

No particular frequency of intercourse is most desirable. Among happy and physically healthy couples, the frequency of intercourse ranges from once a month or less to several times a day. The average frequency, though it should not be interpreted as a goal for an individual couple, is between two and three times a week. A young couple is likely to exceed this frequency, while an older couple would probably engage in intercourse less often.

Problems in Sexual Response

Today increasing numbers of people are seeking professional help for sexual problems. It is doubtful that sexual problems have become more common in recent years, but our expectations and standards for mutually satisfactory relations have definitely risen. Increased openness about sex has led people who would have suffered in silence to seek help. However, many people still do shoulder their troubles alone rather than seek aid. Since sexual adequacy is such an important part of a positive self-concept, it is often difficult or even impossible to admit to a sexual problem. If people realized how common sexual problems are, it might be easier for them to seek the professional help that sexual complaints, like all health problems, require.

Often sexual problems are called *dysfunctions* (the combining form "dys-" means "difficult") to reflect the functional nature of these disorders. There is nothing organically or structurally wrong with the physical organs of sex; they simply are working improperly. When the impediment to normal function is removed, they work again as they should.

Problems in Male Sexuality

The incidence of sexual dysfunction among males is quite high. We will consider some of the more common male complaints.

IMPOTENCE

Impotence is the inability to achieve and/or maintain an erection. While some authorities consider premature ejaculation to be a form of impotence, the authors prefer to follow Masters and Johnson in defining impotence in terms of erectile incompetence and in considering premature ejaculation as a separate problem. This does not preclude the possibility, however, that for many men the two problems coexist and result from the same cause.

Cases of impotence can be classified as either *primary*, in which successful coitus has never been achieved, or *secondary*, in which impotence appears in a previously potent man. As with female dysfunction, the incidence of impotence depends on how you define the term. Only a few men are totally impotent throughout their lives. Much more common is the situation of transient impotence resulting from some temporary emotional problem. On any given day, many men would be suffering from some degree of temporary impotence. In fact, it would be an unusual man who would make it through his entire lifetime without encountering at least a few situations of impotence.

Impotence may be caused by physical (biological) or psychological factors or a combination of the two. The great majority of cases (over 90 percent) are mainly psychological, but before automatically treating impotence as a psychological problem, it is important to rule out any possible physical cause. In general, primary impotence is more often associated with biological factors than is secondary impotence, but either can have biological or psychological causes. In determining cause, it's important to know whether erection ever occurs. Many men who are impotent when attempting coitus with women do have erections at other times, such as while asleep or upon awakening in the morning. (Erection commonly accompanies the rapid eye movement [REM] phase of sleep, which often occurs just prior to awakening in the morning.) Many impotent men are also able to achieve erection and masturbate to orgasm. Such cases of impotence are almost certainly of psychological origin. In contrast, if morning erections seldom or never occur and if erection through masturbation is impossible, then there is a strong probability that a physical factor is causing the impotence. A very few men go through life without ever experiencing an erection. Such cases, called *absolute impotence*, are almost surely of biological origin.

Many physical factors may cause impotence. Fatigue and heavy use of alcohol or other drugs are prime causes. Also, many medications, such as tranquilizers, may cause impotence as a side effect. The possibility of hormonal problems must also be considered. Diabetes is a common hormonal cause of impotence. Insufficient hormone secretion by the pituitary gland (gonadotropic hormones) or the testes (testosterone) will also cause impotence. There may be abnormalities in the sex chromosomes. Certain surgical procedures, such as those necessary in cancers of the prostate or colon, are followed by a high incidence of impotence. The normal aging process is usually associated with some decline in potency, though there is a great variation among men in this respect. In this, as well as in most of the other causes of impotence, a man is likely to develop a great concern over his declining potency, which tends to compound the problem. Ironically, the fear of impotence is one of the most important psychological causes of impotence.

A multitude of psychological factors can act, either singly or in various combinations, to produce impotence. There is no one underlying psychological conflict present in all cases of impotence, nor any impotence-causing conflict that is not also present in many normally potent men.

There is, in the minds of many men, a considerable exaggeration regarding the "inevitable" loss of sexual potency with aging. Millions of men secretly fear that any day their potency will suddenly fail them. The first instance of impotence for a man often occurs at a time when he has been drinking or using other drugs, is under some great temporary emotional stress, or is fatigued. Perhaps he attains an erection, but loses it halfway through coitus or during the preliminary sex play. The next time he attempts coitus, he is probably going to be worried about his potency. Remember that erection of the penis is controlled through the parasympathetic branch of the autonomic nervous system. The autonomic nervous

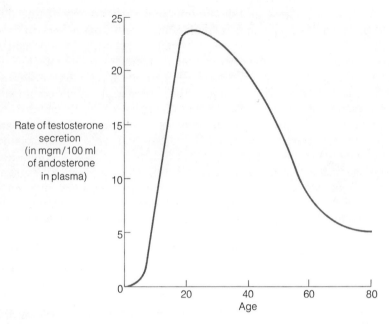

Figure 3.4 *Rate of testosterone secretion in the male, by age. Note peak at age 17-18*

system is not under direct conscious control, but its actions are determined by the emotional state of the individual. The parasympathetic branch is stimulated by a feeling of well-being and inhibited by emotions such as fear, anxiety, or anger. Thus it is quite impossible to attain an erection by conscious will, no matter how much one desires it, if the basic emotional state is such that the parasympathetic nervous system is being inhibited. Thus the fear of failure can set up a cycle that assumes failure.

Other sources of impotence-causing anxiety include fear of being caught in an extramarital affair (may cause impotence with either woman or with both), fear of premature ejaculation, fear of being judged as sexually inferior, fear of causing pregnancy, and fear of venereal disease.

Other psychological causes of impotence include resentment toward the sexual partner, as in the case of a passive man who is dominated by an aggressive wife or the converse situation where a man feels a woman is overly dependent upon him. Impotence is sometimes seen as an unconscious means of "punishing" a woman by denying the fulfillment of her sexual needs. There may be a hostility toward women in general, conscious or unconscious negative feelings or disgust about sex, or a variety of neurotic personality disturbances.

The treatment of impotence resulting from psychological causes varies considerably from therapist to therapist, depending largely on the school of thought to which he belongs. The man and his sexual partner may well be treated as a unit, since impotence often revolves around the complex network of interactions between the two. Regardless of the approach, the goal in treating impotence is to discover the stress-producing factors blocking normal sexual response and then to minimize or eliminate them.

PREMATURE EJACULATION

When is ejaculation premature? Anyone would agree that ejaculation prior to or immediately following vaginal penetration is premature. But what about ejaculation after 2 minutes? After 5 minutes? What about ejaculation after the partner has had one orgasm but would like to have several more? What about a man whose erection can last for 50 minutes, but whose partner needs an hour of intensive coitus to reach her orgasm? Obviously, there can be no clear-cut definition of premature ejaculation. Masters and Johnson (1966) consider a man to have a problem of premature ejaculation if he cannot delay ejaculation long enough to satisfy his *normally* responsive partner in at least 50 percent of their coital experiences. Perhaps ejaculation is best considered premature if it seems so to either sexual partner.

Indeed, premature ejaculation has not always been recognized as a problem. There was a time when a man might have been proud of how quickly he ejaculated, as a supposed sign of great virility. As long as women were not really expected to enjoy coitus, it made little difference how long coitus was sustained.

Very few men are likely to get through life without at least a few instances of "premature" ejaculation. In fact, under certain conditions, premature ejaculation must be considered entirely normal and predictable. For example, it is unrealistic to expect a young man who has been without any sexual release for many days to withhold his ejaculation until his partner has achieved orgasm. Similarly, the first act of coitus with a new and highly exciting woman may be normally expected to result in a "premature" ejaculation.

How then do you distinguish "normal" premature ejaculation from the "problem" variety? The distinction here is that if a man has regular and frequent intercourse with the same woman that often ends in premature ejaculation, it is a problem. In such a case, the underlying psychological causes may be quite similar to those causing impotence. Examples include: hostility toward the woman, where premature ejaculation is used to deny her sexual satisfaction; guilt about sex, in which premature ejaculation is used to deny her sexual satisfaction; guilt about sex, in which premature ejaculation helps to "get it over with"; feelings of sexual inadequacy, in which there is a rush to prove that the penis is still "working"; fears; and love conflicts.

Ejaculation, like erection, is controlled through the autonomic branch of the nervous system. Thus ejaculation cannot be controlled by direct conscious effort. While erection is inhibited by the sympathetic branch, ejaculation is promoted by it. Thus the stress that can produce impotence may also result in premature ejaculation. In fact, the two problems often exist in the same individual.

As in impotence, the reaction of a man's sexual partner greatly influences his chances of overcoming premature ejaculation. If she ridicules or chastises him, he is in trouble. If she reassures him and minimizes the problem, then he has a very good chance of overcoming it.

There is no shortage of advice for the man who is bothered by premature ejaculation. For persistent premature ejaculation, there should be, first of all, a physical examination for such physical causes as urethritis, prostatitis, cystitis (bladder infection), and diabetes. If no physical cause can be found, then psychotherapy is often recommended. As with impotence, the regular sexual partner may well be included in the therapeutic process. Masters and Johnson, in the book *Human Sexual Inadequacy,* take a more directly physical approach, recommending an "exercise" for premature ejaculation in which the woman's hand stimulates the man's penis almost to the point of orgasm, then, with the thumb and fingers tightly squeezes the base of the glans penis. Done repeatedly, as detailed in their book, this technique often solves long-term problems of premature ejaculation.

If premature ejaculation occurs in one of the "normal" situations described above, then the male is likely to be so highly aroused that a second erection can be attained in a few minutes and, with seminal pressure reduced, prolonged intercourse should be possible. If premature ejaculation occurs repeatedly in second and subsequent erections, then the premature ejaculation is of the "problem" type, and professional counsel should be sought. Also, in many cases, reerection after premature ejaculation is impossible, even in a young man who should be capable of a second erection, illustrating the close relationship between premature ejaculation and impotence.

Many other suggestions are offered for the prevention of premature ejaculation. These would be of value only in cases where there is no serious underlying psychological cause. Some physicians prescribe mild tranquilizers for their patients who complain of premature ejaculation. Some doctors recommend that an anesthetic ointment be applied over the glans of the penis to reduce the sensory stimulus. A similar effect can sometimes be obtained by wearing a condom (rubber). Regular sex partners can learn to prolong coitus by holding very still for a few seconds whenever ejaculation seems imminent. Some men learn to fantasize about nonsexual objects when ejaculation is imminent. Premature ejaculation is sometimes associated with inadequate foreplay and with penetration of the vagina while it is still poorly lubricated and tight; the increased friction makes control difficult. Through experimenting with different coital positions, a couple may find one or more in which ejaculatory control is improved. Positions with the woman lying, sitting, or kneeling over the man are sometimes helpful. Though professional help may be necessary, premature ejaculation can almost always be remedied.

RETARDED EJACULATION

Much less common than premature ejaculation, but certainly not rare, is its opposite—retarded ejaculation. In some men, ejaculation occurs only with great effort, or not at all. In coitus (or masturbation), such a man may struggle to ejaculate until he exhausts himself and, perhaps, his sexual partner. Coitus is usually accompanied by emotional withdrawal and reduced sexual sensations. The man senses emotional detachment from his partner and feels as if his penis were anesthetized.

Retarded ejaculation may occur when the male is very tired and doesn't have the ready energy required for ejaculation. It may also be due to damage to the nerves controlling ejaculation. Usually, however, it is the result of psychological causes, often associated with a paranoid tendency. Two factors characteristic of paranoid males seem to produce this symptom. One is an excessive concern with masculinity, derived from an ever-present fear of being forced into submission by a more dominant female. The other is the "paranoid rage," a strong impulse to commit violence. Since ejaculation results in loss of erection, it can be seen as a threat to masculinity. This threat triggers the rage, which acts through the autonomic nervous system to prevent ejaculation.

Persistent retarded ejaculation is usually treated through psychotherapy, where the goal is to reduce the patient's tremendous concern with his masculinity and his accompanying fear and rage.

PENIS ANXIETIES

Many young men suffer needless anxiety about the size of the penis. Some worry that it may be too small to satisfy a woman; some fear that it may be too large to fit into the vagina. All of these fears are needless. The size of the penis and, further, whether or not it is circumcised have nothing to do with the sexual satisfaction of the man himself or of the woman. Sexual technique and experience are the important things.

The diameter of the vagina stretches to fit the size of the penis. Even after several babies have been born, the vagina usually remains small enough in diameter to tightly contain even the smallest penis. On the other hand, the vagina is capable of stretching enough to allow the passage of a baby, so a large penis will certainly create no problem.

As far as length of penis is concerned, very few sensory receptors are found in the deeper part of the vagina. Such receptors are concentrated on the clitoris and labia and outer vagina. As a result, it is difficult or impossible for a woman to feel the difference between a long penis and a short one.

Some young men even worry about the fact that their penis seems to curve (most do curve) or have some other irregularity. Every man should realize that the size or shape of the penis is of negligible importance in sexual intercourse.

Problems in Female Sexuality

Some of the more common forms of female sexual dysfunction include hyporesponsiveness ("lack of interest" in sex), difficulty in attaining orgasm, and painful coitus. While these symptoms might seem to indicate totally different types of problems, their underlying causes are often quite similar.

Since female dysfunction is defined in various ways, statistics on its incidence vary with the meaning given the word. Most of the studies on sexual response have concentrated on married women, thus ignoring any women who might have remained single because of their hyporesponsiveness. Another variable is the basis of the survey. Some have been based on how often coitus is desired, some on how often it actually occurs, and some on how often orgasm is reached in coitus, or from all types of stimulation. In any case, it seems that sexual hyporesponsiveness is a constant problem for many women (perhaps 15 or 20 percent), while transient or situational dysfunction in response to temporary conditions would occur at some time during the life of almost every woman.

Sexual dysfunction may affect a woman's relationships with men. It may, in its more severe forms, influence even her nonsexual relationships, especially if her problem is associated with a fear or resentment of men. The effects of dysfunction on marriage are usually obvious and predictable. The husband will feel angry, unloved, rejected, and sexually inadequate and might, as an ego defense, become involved in extramarital affairs in order to confirm his own sexual adequacy. The effects on the woman herself are difficult to separate from the psychological characteristics likely to underlie her dysfunction. Sexual dysfunction is usually the cause, as well as the effect, of emotional problems. Traits often associated with dysfunction, either as cause or effect, are anxiety, depression, tension, frustration, general unhappiness, and a multitude of psychosomatic complaints. Any direct physical effects would occur mainly in the woman who is sexually responsive and becomes highly aroused for long periods of time, but without the relief of orgasm. In such cases, the pelvic blood vessels remain dilated and a painful pelvic congestion may result.

Problems in female sexual response are generally due to psychological rather than physical causes. The basic biological drive and capacity for sexual satisfaction is present, but is blocked by psychological factors acting on the sympathetic nervous system. Some cases, however, are in fact caused by biological factors, such as hormone imbalance. A first step for any woman concerned with her sexual response should be a complete physical to find or rule out any possible biological causes of her problem.

Many psychological factors are implicated in dysfunction. Fear often causes inadequate female response. There may be a fear of men, fear of the penis, fear of pregnancy, fear of venereal disease, fear of physical or emotional hurt, fear of loss of identity, or fear of being physically or emotionally close to someone. Hostility is another obstacle to female response. It may be hostility toward men in general or toward a specific man. Many women respond very differently with different partners. Many daughters of strictly moralistic parents are left with a persistent feeling that sex is wrong, and their guilt may inhibit them.

A previously responsive woman may become unresponsive after being emotionally hurt a few times in her relationships with men. As an ego defense she learns to avoid full emotional commitment for fear that she might once again be disappointed and hurt. Similarly, a woman who was emotionally deprived as a child, raised by perhaps cold and unloving parents, may as an adult find herself unable to take the risk of disappointment inherent in any close interpersonal relationship. In either case, the woman consciously or unconsciously decides that, rather than loving a man and taking the chance of his rejecting her, she will reject him first. Such a woman may be very independent in all aspects of her life, driven to perform in school, in a career, and perhaps in sports. She may be successful by most objective measures of success, but in many cases seems never really very happy.

The male's role in causing female dysfunction deserves further emphasis. Many men are really directly responsible for their partner's unresponsiveness. Some men never display any trace of love or attention to the woman, then cannot understand why she is not instantly aroused when they want sex. Other men are so sexually inhibited that they in turn destroy their partner's potential for enjoyment. Their inhibition may prevent them from adequately arousing the woman with precoital sex play and may also lead to premature ejaculation. After enough instances of premature ejaculation, a woman often finds that she would rather not bother to risk further disappointment and becomes unresponsive.

Compulsive Sexuality

Common among both sexes are people whose sex lives consist of an endless series of brief encounters with ever-changing partners. Seldom is any level of emotional intimacy established, and there is often a hollow or "something-is-missing" feeling. Although these people may engage in seemingly normal intercourse quite frequently, they often gain no emotional satisfaction from it.

In males, this problem is sometimes called the *Don Juan complex*—if the emphasis is on the number of different sexual partners—or *satyriasis*—if the emphasis is on the frequency of sexual contact. The term *nymphomaniac* is sometimes applied to women who seem to have unusually high numbers of heterosexual encounters.

Several personality traits are commonly associated with compulsive sexuality. The foremost is probably a feeling (which can be unconscious) of sexual or personal inadequacy. The person needs to constantly "prove" his or her ability to attract lovers and function sexually. But regardless of the number of lovers attracted or orgasms reached, the fear of inadequacy remains.

Fear of intimacy is also common. Many people, perhaps as a result of past emotional hurts or their feelings of inadequacy, lack the confidence required to establish a close relationship with another person. Lacking intimacy, their sexual relationships always seem incomplete, so the search for satisfaction must continue.

Many people have been raised in sexually repressive atmospheres. Sexual guilt or inhibition, perhaps as a result of childhood conditioning, may act to deny sexual satisfaction, even though full physiological orgasm may occur.

Finally, compulsive sexuality may be a part of a broader antisocial or sociopathic personality. Someone with an antisocial personality is unable to postpone immediate pleasure or gratification of an impulse, lacks the capacity for maintaining a close relationship with another person, and feels no guilt or anxiety over antisocial acts. Such a person would probably have a history of job problems and regular run-ins with the law in addition to compulsive sexuality.

Like other forms of sexual dysfunction, compulsive sexuality can often be treated successfully by a qualified therapist. Treatment may involve building a sense of personal or sexual adequacy, developing the ability to establish intimacy with another person, or extinguishing feelings of guilt or inhibition. People with antisocial personalities generally require more basic therapy since their compulsive sexuality is just one symptom of a larger personality disorder.

Treatment of Dysfunction

Since sexual problems most often have psychological causes, treatment usually involves psychotherapy, counseling, or behavior therapy. Hormones or other medications are seldom effective. However, a logical and important first step is a thorough check-up to detect any possible underlying physical causes.

If no physical problem is apparent, consultation should be made with a well-qualified therapist (psychiatrist, clinical psychologist, or marriage counselor). Since the selection of therapists is critical and there are many poorly qualified individuals in this field, it is advisable to obtain a referral or recommendation from a family physician or other health professional. Many cities and towns have tax- or charity-supported family-counseling clinics that treat sexual dysfunction.

A traditional approach to treating sexual problems is psychoanalysis (an extensive probing of the unconscious mind), but this process is often slow and expensive, and the results may be disappointing. The needs of the majority of patients are probably better met through nonpsychoanalytic methods. One approach is to attempt to correct faulty attitudes about sexuality by replacing inhibiting attitudes with more positive feelings. Since the attitudes of both partners are important, the man and the woman are likely to be brought into the therapeutic situation together. Inasmuch as a lack of communication often plays into sexual complaints, therapy may serve as an important way for the partners to learn to express their preferences and inhibitions openly. Behavior therapy, based on the idea that behavior is determined by modifiable stimulus-response patterns, centers around the reconditioning of responses to given stimuli, with the goal of developing more appropriate responses. It is often quite successful.

Summary

I. Sexual Stimuli

    A. People respond to a variety of stimuli

    B. Both sexes respond to about the same stimuli

II. Male Sexual Response

    A. Excitement—erection of the penis by engorgement with blood under control of autonomic nervous system

    B. Plateau

        1. Erect penis increases in diameter

        2. Preejaculatory fluid is emitted

        3. Testes elevate and enlarge

        4. Sex flush appears, breathing and heart rates increase, muscular tension develops over body

    C. Orgasm

        1. Ejaculation of semen

        2. Ejaculation during sleep is nocturnal emission

    D. Resolution

        1. Penis usually loses erection

        2. Minimum interval before repeated erection may vary from minutes to days

III. Female Sexual Response

    A. Excitement

        1. Clitoris increases in length, labia spread

        2. Vagina lubricates and lengthens

    B. Plateau

        1. Clitoris moves under its hood

        2. Labia swell and turn bright red

    C. Orgasm—series of contractions of uterus and vagina

D. Resolution—sex organs return to normal size

E. Time needed to reach orgasm varies

F. Intensity and duration of orgasm vary

G. Many women are capable of multiple orgasms

H. Very few women reach orgasm in every instance of sexual intercourse

IV. The Nervous System and Sexual Response

   A. Autonomic (involuntary) system controls sexual response

   B. Autonomic system has two subdivisions:

      1. Parasympathetic branch

         a. Activated by sense of well-being

         b. Stimulates sexual arousal

      2. Sympathetic branch

         a. Activated by fear, anger, worry, anxiety, hostility, and similar emotions

         b. Inhibits sexual arousal

V. Sexual Techniques

   A. Open couple-communication of sexual likes and dislikes is very important

   B. Before intercourse—adequate sex play helps prepare both partners

   C. Sexual intercourse—any mutually enjoyable position is fine

VI. Frequency of Intercourse

   A. A source of conflict in many relationships

   B. No particular frequency is most desirable

VII. Problems in Sexual Response

   A. Term dysfunction reflects functional (nonorganic) nature of most sexual problems

   B. Problems in male sexuality

      1. Impotence

         a. Inability to achieve or maintain erection

         b. Causes may be physical, psychological, or a combination of the two

         c. Great majority of cases are psychological

         d. Physical causes include excessive use of alcohol or other drugs, fatigue, side effect of medication, diabetes, other hormonal problems, certain surgical procedures

         e. Multitude of psychological factors may be involved

f. Can include anything that activates sympathetic branch of nervous system

g. Fear of impotence is a common cause

h. Treatment similar to treatment of female dysfunction

2. Premature ejaculation

   a. No clear definition

   b. Should be expected under certain circumstances

   c. Considered a problem when same man and woman have regular sex and man frequently ejaculates before normally responsive woman is satisfied

   d. Ejaculation controlled by sympathetic branch of autonomic nervous system

   e. Thus caused by same emotional factors that produce impotence

   f. Many approaches to treatment are discussed

3. Retarded ejaculation

   a. Less common than premature ejaculation, but not rare

   b. Almost always has psychological causes

4. Penis anxieties

   a. Many men worry about size of penis

   b. Size of penis not important to sexual satisfaction of man or woman

   c. Technique and experience are the important things

C. Problems in female sexuality

1. Common forms of female dysfunction include hyporesponsiveness, difficulty in attaining orgasm, and painful coitus

2. Causes of female dysfunction

   a. Usually psychological, rather than physical

   b. Normal sexual response is blocked by activation of sympathetic branch of autonomic nervous system

   c. Could involve fear, hostility, guilt, conflicting loves

   d. Male often causes female hyporesponsiveness through his inattention, inhibition, or poor techniques

D. Compulsive sexuality

1. Characterized by series of brief sexual encounters without intimacy

2. Associated personality traits may include:

   a. Feeling of sexual or total personal inadequacy

      b. Fear of intimacy

      c. Sexual inhibition or guilt

      d. Antisocial (sociopathic) personality development

  E. Treatment of dysfunction

      1. Usually involves psychotherapy, counseling, or behavior therapy

      2. Should first check for physical causes

      3. Must select therapist carefully—many quacks in this field

      4. Should include usual sexual partner in therapy

Questions for Review

1. What factors have tended to prevent objective research on sex?

2. Describe the stages in male and female sexual response.

3. In what ways do male and female sexual responses differ?

4. Should a woman expect to reach orgasm every time she makes love?

5. In what ways have expectations for sexual satisfaction and performance changed in the past 50 years?

6. What position should a couple use for their lovemaking?

7. Summarize the relationship between the autonomic nervous system and sexual problems.

8. What are some of the causes of sexual dysfunction?

9. Should premature ejaculation be considered a type of impotence?

10. Outline the causes of impotence.

11. When is an ejaculation "premature"?

12. What are some common causes of compulsive sexuality?

13. Outline an approach to the treatment of sexual dysfunction.

14. Why should the sexual partner be included in the treatment of sexual problems?

Chapter 4
VARIATIONS IN SEXUAL EXPRESSION

Sexual behavior, like all human action, is motivated by the needs of the individual. These needs, in turn, result from inherent biological and emotional characteristics modified and developed through a lifetime of experience, observation, and interpretation. Since each of us lives an essentially different life, it is not surprising that our needs and sexual behaviors likewise differ.

With the exception of solitary masturbation, sexual behavior involves other people. Thus sexual needs and actions take on a social dimension. When an individual's activity runs up against the expectations and behavior preferred by his culture, the person may find himself enmeshed in social and even legal conflicts. Some of society's greatest contemporary controversies concern the definition of acceptable sexual behavior. While certain actions, such as forcible rape, are condemned by almost everyone, others, such as prostitution and homosexual love between consenting adults, seem permissible to some and reprehensible to others.

In this chapter, we will look at sexual variations and at the dilemmas they occasion for the individual and for society.

Homosexuality

Most prominent of the sexual variations—both in the attention of behavioral scientists and in the news media—is *homosexuality*, sexual relationships with members of one's own sex. Almost all aspects of homosexuality are controversial, but certain facts seem fairly well substantiated.

Different authorities give divergent estimates of the incidence of homosexuality in the American population. However, it appears that between 4 to 10 percent of our adult population is exclusively homosexual. A much larger group, variously estimated at between 25 to 50 percent of both males and females passes through a period of transient homosexual feeling and/or activity during the preadolescent or adolescent years before becoming exclusively heterosexual.

It appears that the number of *bisexuals*, people who enjoy sexual relations with both males and females, is growing, particularly in the more cosmopolitan areas of the United States and Europe. The number of bisexuals is now believed to exceed the number of homosexuals. The causes of this phenomenon are not yet truly understood.

Apparently sexual orientation may lie anywhere along a continuum ranging from exclusive homosexuality to exclusive heterosexuality. Many people have developed sexual lifestyles that fall somewhere between these two.

Patterns of Homosexual Behavior

Despite the more extreme images popularized in recent years, homosexuals are seldom noticeably different in dress, speech, or other behavior from the heterosexual majority. The few male homosexuals who do display their sexual orientation may adopt either effeminate mode of dress and action or a supermasculine image, with well-developed muscles, leather clothing, motorcycles, or similar symbols of stereotyped masculinity. Female homosexuals (*lesbians*) may similarly range in appearance from masculine to extremely feminine.

The typical pattern of homosexual relationships differs considerably between males and females. The male tendency is to seek more variety in sexual partners. Long-term, exclusive relationships are less common among male homosexuals. Instead, the male homosexual often searches constantly for new sexual encounters, cruising gay bars and similar homosexual gathering places. Since current laws make homosexuality illegal, the male homosexual openly seeking a partner runs a steady risk of arrest. He is also exposed to the possibility of venereal disease, harrassment, and occasionally blackmail.

Among lesbians, long-term relationships are quite common, many lasting years or a lifetime. In these relationships, one member sometimes assumes a more dominant, masculine role in both dress and actions, while the other partner assumes a feminine role. However, these roles are by no means typical of all lesbian arrangements.

Among the practices used by male homosexuals to achieve orgasm are mutual hand manipulation of the penis, oral–genital contact, and anal–genital contact. Techniques used in female homosexual contacts include kissing, manual and oral manipulation of the breasts, and manual or oral stimulation of the genitals.

Some homosexuals enter into heterosexual marriages for any of a number of reasons. Sometimes the individual is truly bisexual and enjoys relationships with both sexes. More often, the marriage is the homosexual's attempt to live a "straight" life, thinking that marriage may overcome homosexuality (it seldom does). Or marriage can be a "front" for homosexual activity, a ruse to appear socially acceptable while privately engaging in homosexual activities. The mates chosen for these marriages are often individuals with low sex drives who make few heterosexual demands on the homosexual.

Causes of Homosexuality

There is very little evidence to support a biological theory of homosexuality. While a few studies have shown minor hormonal differences between homosexual and heterosexual men, most authorities regard homosexuality as an emotional phenomenon. It is a mistake to overgeneralize when describing the causes of homosexuality, for they are numerous, psychologically complex, and different from person to person. However, it is generally agreed that the influences leading to homosexuality usually arise during childhood. In fact, homosexuality or heterosexuality is usually so strongly determined by the time the individual is 20 years old that, without therapy, the chance of a change in sexual orientation after that time is remote.

The relationship between the child and his parents often contributes to the development of homosexuality. Failure to identify with the parent of the same sex is common among homosexuals. The homosexual male is often found to have had an unusually strong attachment to his mother or sister. Homosexuality may also arise in the case of a child who realizes that his sex disappointed one or both of his parents, especially if their disappointment leads them to treat the child as if he were of the opposite sex.

The causes of female homosexuality are apparently even more diverse and often more subtle than those of male homosexuality. It is not generally the case that girls become lesbians as a result of overly close attachment to their fathers. Actually, most girls who have close relationships with their fathers remain strongly heterosexual. Lesbians typically report disruptive and unstable family backgrounds and poor relationships with either or both parents. Various emotionally traumatic experiences have typically led to a deep sense of insecurity and inadequacy, a belief that they cannot get along well with males, a distrust of males, and strong prejudices against (or fears of) male-female relationships.

Isolated incidents of homosexual behavior can result from temporary needs and drives rather than from any deeply rooted homosexual attitudes. Sexual play between children of the same sex is common and does not usually lead to any adult homosexuality. Occasional episodes of homosexual experimentation in adolescence do not necessarily mean that the individuals will become homosexual adults. Even adults, when isolated from the opposite sex, as in prison or the military, may engage in homosexual activities without being regarded as true homosexuals. The same may be true of isolated cases of homosexual behavior while under the influence of alcohol or other drugs.

Viewpoints on Homosexuality

By no means does everyone see homosexuality as an illness or abnormality. Many homosexuals view their orientation merely as an alternate lifestyle, presenting them with no more difficulties than the typical heterosexual person encounters. Homosexuality meets with varying responses from academics and professionals. Psychiatrists and other physicians, for example, disagree greatly on how to regard homosexuality. Is it an illness, a maladjustment, a neurosis, or an alternative lifestyle? Should treatment be suggested for homosexuality in itself, or should treatment be considered only if a patient's homosexuality is creating problems? In the latter case, should the goal of treatment be to reorient the patient sexually or merely to help him adjust to his homosexuality and its associated problems? There are no clear answers to these questions, and controversy continues to rage in many medical and psychiatric journals. In a significant recent move that may presage the future, the prestigious American Psychiatric Association dropped homosexuality from its list of mental disturbances.

On the other hand, as many as 80 percent of people in the general population consider homosexuality wrong. Typically, better educated city-dwellers of the east and west coasts are more likely to accept it than are less educated rural people.

The law's response to homosexuality is now being critically examined. The simplistic assumption that homosexuality is strictly a legal question, calling for arrest and imprisonment, is clearly being put aside. The professional composition of the National Institute of Mental Health's Task Force on Homosexuality, which published its final report in 1972, indicates the recognized complexity of the problem: the commission included social historians, sociologists, psychologists, judges, and lawyers.

Across the United States, larger communities are currently considering legislation to outlaw discrimination against homosexuals in housing, employment, as well as other denials of civil rights based on sexual preference. Within the next several years, it is likely that tensions between the heterosexual and homosexual communities will continue to ease. This trend has been heralded by the Institute for Sex Research of the University of Indiana, founded originally by Alfred Kinsey in the 1950s. Preliminary results of the Institute's massive study of homosexuality indicate that homosexuals are more and more interested in coming "out of the closet" and into the open to assume the equal place in society so long denied them.

Treatment of Homosexuality

Many psychiatrists and psychologists do see homosexuality as a problem and the homosexual as a person who often displays anxiety, depression, guilt, and irrational jealousies. Although the homosexual can achieve happiness and self-fulfillment, the heterosexual generally finds fewer stumbling blocks in his way.

Perhaps the classification of homosexuality as either a disorder or a lifestyle should depend on the degree of satisfaction and fulfillment the individual homosexual finds in his own life. If the homosexual life is productive and personally fulfilling, there is no obvious rationale for attempting the difficult transition to heterosexuality. If, on the other hand, the individual homosexual is unhappy, hyperanxious, depressed, or dissatisfied with his homosexuality, then it should rightfully be classified as a problem for which he should seek treatment.

As we said above, homosexuality has emotional rather than physical causes and treatment therefore revolves around psychotherapy. Homosexuality has not been treated as successfully as many other types of emotional problems. There are two essential requirements for success. The first is that the homosexual patient must really want to change to a heterosexual life. The second is a therapist who understands homosexuality and is experienced in treating it.

The therapeutic approaches used in treating homosexuality are as varied as the theories explaining the cause of the problem. For example, Freudian psychiatrists use classical psychoanalysis, while behavior therapists employ techniques of positive or aversive conditioning.

Transsexuality

Transsexuality is the conscious, compelling desire to change one's sex. The transsexual feels he or she belongs to the sex opposite to the one that is anatomically apparent. A transsexual thinks, feels, and acts like a person of the opposite sex. He or she may feel trapped in a body of the wrong sex, and sometimes wears the clothing of the desired sex.

Transsexuality is often confused with transvestism (wearing clothing of the opposite sex) and homosexuality. Although both transvestites and many transsexuals dress up like the opposite sex, transvestites are not transsexuals. Similarly, passive homosexuality in the male transsexual is common. However, most homosexuals have a normal gender role; they feel themselves to be true males, not females caught in a male body. The male homosexual enjoys his penis as well as the interest other homosexuals have in it; he derives genital pleasure from his sexual contacts. The transsexual male, on the contrary, hates his penis and derives no pleasure from it at all. Usually he does not experience erection or ejaculation.

The transsexual is usually a biologically normal male or female. With rare exceptions, there are no anatomical, chromosomal, or hormonal abnormalities. Transsexual attitudes can usually be traced back to a childhood background of parents whose sexual roles were unclear or who were disappointed that the child was not of the opposite sex.

Psychotherapy has not been highly successful in the treatment of adult transsexuals, though it is obviously preferable to more radical treatment. Many transsexuals have achieved happiness only after surgical and hormonal sex change procedures. While this is undeniably an extreme measure, the alternatives for many transsexuals are continued suffering or even suicide. Several ethical sex change clinics have been established within the United States, and the majority of their patients have expressed satisfaction with their sex changes. Those changing from male to female (the more common procedure) may be provided with breasts and a vagina, and they may experience sexual pleasure and even orgasm. In the reverse change, it has not been possible to construct an erectile penis, but an artificial penis might be worn for coitus. Of course, natural parenthood is impossible after either sex-change procedure.

Deviate Sexual Behavior

With a few exceptions, our concept of deviate sexuality depends on the context in which specific behavior occurs as well as on the details of the act itself. For example, if a truck driver eating at a diner pinches the waitress, she will very likely wink at him and forget the incident immediately. If a man pinches an attractive but unknown woman on the street, she is apt to call a policeman and have him arrested. As another example, if a man peeks through a bedroom window at a partially dressed woman, he may be arrested and convicted of a sex offense. But looking at even more scantily clothed women in a nightclub act is perfectly acceptable to many members of our society.

Our definition of deviance also includes the psychological component. Specific patterns of deviant sexual behavior can be readily associated with particular mental illnesses and poor social adjustment. The most common forms of deviate sexuality can be discussed in terms of four types of psychopathology: (1) feelings of sexual inferiority, (2) mental incompetence, (3) developmental abnormalities, and (4) a disposition towards violence.

Sexual Insecurity

The fear of sexual inadequacy can be associated with certain types of deviance. For any one of a number of reasons, the sexually insecure person has been made to feel ashamed or disgraced because of a real or imagined inability to function satisfactorily in heterosexual relationships. From this single foundation, a variety of deviate behavior patterns can arise.

EXHIBITIONISM

Exhibitionism is the purposeful exposure of the penis to an unsuspecting female without any intention of further sexual contact. Apparently, the exhibitionist's intention is to arouse an emotional expression in the victim. Because of the underlying sexual inferiority complex associated with exhibitionism, the desired response is shock at the size of the exhibitionist's sex organs. An amused reaction can be extremely crushing. Most exhibitionists are harmless, and there is seldom if ever a danger of rape. In most cases, the safest and best response for a woman encountering an exhibitionist is merely to ignore him.

OBSCENE PHONE CALLS

Obscene phone calls are anonymous communication with a female without intention of further sexual contact. Like the exhibitionist, the obscene phone-caller finds sexual release in the act itself or in masturbation during the call. The hoped-for reaction is shock and consternation on the part of the victim. The fact that the victim is both inaccessible and unknown protects the deviate from a possible sexual confrontation. The best way to deal with an obscene phone call is for the woman simply to hang up. The longer she stays on the phone, the more she is likely to encourage the deviate. If she transmits fear or shock, she is playing his game and inviting further calls.

VOYEURISM

Voyeurism is obtaining sexual gratification by looking at sexual objects or situations. This is probably the most difficult sexual deviation to isolate. Almost all people have some voyeuristic tendencies, and enjoy nude shows in bars, reading sophisticated magazines, and watching attractive people in brief bathing suits. The "peeping Tom" is gratified by seeing females nude or partially nude without their knowledge or consent. He often masturbates while peeping. A few peepers call attention to themselves by actions such as tapping on a window, but the vast majority of peepers try to avoid detection. The peeper is generally shy with women, and despite a heterosexual orientation, reluctant to seek normal relationships with them. Like the exhibitionist and the obscene phone-caller, the peeper is usually harmless.

Mental Incompetence

Some sexual deviations result from mental inadequacy. The two examples discussed below are generally associated with rural communities and undereducated individuals.

BESTIALITY

Bestiality is sexual contact with animals. This is apparently a common occurrence among rural boys, yet bestiality is one of the most taboo forms of sexual conduct. Even in rural areas, it is the object of both condemnation and ridicule. Bestiality is usually not an end in itself but only a substitute for

more normal sexual relationships. The animal is used as an aid to masturbation, rather than as a true sexual stimulus.

INCEST

Incest is sexual relationships between two people too closely related to
marry legally. The relationship can be father-daughter, father-
stepdaughter, mother-son, mother-stepson, or brother-sister. Incest is one
of the most ancient and widespread of the sexual taboos. Most incidents of
incest develop either within a subculture that takes a less strict attitude
toward such behavior or as a result of the mental incompetence of one of
the partners. Even in the contemporary United States, there remain certain
subcultures in which incest is thought of as unfortunate, but not a grave or
unexpected situation. Gebhard et al. (1965) found that incest is most
common among impoverished, unintelligent, uneducated individuals living in rural surroundings. They come from a cultural background wherein
sexual morality is publicly emphasized, but privately breached with im-
punity.

Developmental Abnormalities

Some forms of sexual deviance are associated with the failure of the
individual to develop normally. Either because of an inability to attain
normal sexual maturity or because of a regression (return) to earlier,
immature sexual habits, this type of deviate is likely to show one of the
following behavior patterns.

PEDOPHILIA

Pedophilia is sexual involvement of an adult with a child. It may take either
heterosexual or homosexual forms. With the exception of incest,
pedophilia is probably the least acceptable sexual deviance in our society.
Since the deviation lies in the sexual immaturity of the child, the natural
break-off point for classifying an act as pedophilia would be the onset of
puberty. Pedophiles are usually characterized psychologically as suffering
from an arrested development (fixation) in which the offender has never
grown psychosexually beyond the immature prepubertal stage, or from a
regression back to this stage of development. As a result, the great majority
of sexual acts in pedophilia consist of the sex-play type found in children,
such as looking, showing, fondling, and being fondled. The nature of the
sexual act usually corresponds to the maturity expected at the age of the
victim rather than at the age of the offender. Research has shown that the
social aftereffects of a molestation incident can be much more devastating
to the child than the incident itself.

FETISHISM

Fetishism is sexual stimulation from perception and possession of inani-
mate objects. The heterosexual development of the fetishist is generally

poor. Fetishism is a displacement reaction, a sexual response not to a living object, but to a symbol of that object. A certain amount of fetishism is entirely normal. Certain items of clothing, such as black lace panties, have so universally been equated with sex appeal that some sexual arousal from the sight of them is neither surprising nor abnormal. At what point, then, does a fetish become abnormal? Some possible criteria for fetishism include: when the sexual arousal from the fetish item is frequently strong enough to cause erection; when the fetish item is often used in masturbation; when the fetish item is necessary for erection for intercourse; when sexual partners are chosen on the basis of possession of the fetish item; when the fetish item is collected (through purchase or theft).

TRANSVESTISM

Transvestism is the wearing of clothing of the opposite sex. Transvestism is a complex phenomenon, with more than one root cause. Some transvestites are homosexuals and wear garments of the opposite sex as an outward sign of homosexuality (to attract persons of the same sex) and as a symbol of the wearer's preferred role in homosexual acts. The "true" transvestite, on the other hand, wears the clothing of the opposite sex for the emotional or sexual gratification it provides. This type of transvestism is an end in itself, not just advertising for sex partners.

Violent Behavior

A disposition towards unnecessary violence and an orientation to use force to deal with emotional needs and desires is the basis of certain types of deviant sexual patterns. For this reason, these deviances pose the very real danger of physical harm.

FORCIBLE RAPE

Forcible rape is the use of violence to force a female to submit to sexual intercourse. A detailed study of men convicted of forcible rape (Gebhard et al., 1965) indicated that they fall into several distinct groups. The most common type of rapist was a man whose entire way of life includes the use of unnecessary violence. This type of rapist does not commit rape because of a lack of willing sex partners. Instead, he prefers rape to conventional sex. Rapists often have underlying inferiority feelings, and a sense of dominance is compulsively important to them. For this type of individual, sexual intercourse is most gratifying only if it is accompanied by physical violence or the serious threat of violence. This indicates a strong sadistic element in the personality of this most common type of rapist; he dislikes women and gains satisfaction from punishing them. Often more violence is used than necessary to complete the rape. In some cases, the violence seems to substitute for sexual release or at least to diminish the need for it. In fact, these rapists sometimes become impotent and are unable to culminate the sex attack.

A second type of rapist is the amoral delinquent. These men pay little attention to normal social controls and operate purely for their own gratification. They are not sadistic—they simply want to have intercourse, and the contrary wishes of the female are of no importance. They are not hostile toward females, but look upon them solely as sexual objects whose role in life is to provide sexual pleasure to men.

A third type of rapist is the drunken variety. The drunk's aggression ranges from uncoordinated efforts at seduction to hostile and truly vicious behavior released by the lowering of inhibitions due to intoxication.

A fourth type of rapist is the "explosive" variety. These are previously normal individuals who have suddenly snapped into a psychotic state as a result of emotional stresses. An example might be a mild-natured college student who suddenly rapes and kills.

A woman can best reduce her chances of being a victim by avoiding those situations that most often lead to forcible rape. Of these, touring bars alone is the most frequently mentioned by women who report forcible rape. (Incidentally, many rapes are never reported, owing to embarrassment, fear of retaliation, or desire to avoid courtroom cross-examination.) Hitching rides is another good way to meet a rapist. Among young girls, running away from home often leads to rape.

There can be no clear answer to the question of what to do when faced with a rapist. This question can be answered only on the spot, since circumstances can vary so much. Among approaches that sometimes work are calmly talking the rapist into changing his mind, making lots of noise, or tricking him in one way or another. But even the best planned defense may fall apart in the suddenness and fear of the actual attack. A rapist can be extremely dangerous. Distasteful as it sounds, if rape seems unavoidable, it is highly advisable for the woman to yield to and cooperate with her assailant; it is far better to be raped and alive than raped and dead.

SADISM

Sadism is attaining sexual satisfaction by inflicting cruelty on another person. The sexual sadist is often unable to achieve orgasm without the use of some form of violence. There are both male and female sadists and both heterosexual and homosexual sadism. As we mentioned in the discussion of forcible rape, sadism is often a motivating factor in rape. The rapist frequently uses more force than necessary to complete the rape, and elements of torture are sometimes involved. Many men use sadistic cruelty in their relationships with prostitutes or even with their wives, being unable to gain satisfaction without this cruelty. Sadism can take forms apparently unrelated to its sexual basis. According to some authorities, such forms of violence as child-beating, wife-beating, and professional boxing have a sadistic basis.

MASOCHISM

Masochism is the attainment of sexual gratification from suffering physical pain. There are both men and women who must be physically punished in order to gain sexual arousal or orgasm. The punishment often involves beating, whipping, biting, pinching, scratching, burning, and similar painful treatments. Various psychological explanations have been offered for masochism. It has been interpreted in terms of the destructive impulses carried in the unconscious mind. It has also been related to subconscious guilt feelings temporarily relieved by the masochistic punishment.

Summary

I. Homosexualtiy

    A. Sexual attraction to members of same sex

    B. Estimated 4 to 10 percent of men and women are exclusively homosexual

    C. Many more people are bisexual—attracted to both sexes

    D. Most homosexuals cannot be recognized by appearance

    E. Homosexual behavior patterns

        1. Females (lesbians) tend to form more lasting relationships than do males

        2. Various manual, oral, anal, and genital practices used in homosexual lovemaking

    F. Causes of homosexuality

        1. Most authorities cite psychological rather than biological causes

        2. Often attributed to parent-child and parent-parent relationships during early childhood

        3. Difficult or impossible to pinpoint causes for specific individuals

    G. Viewpoints on homosexuality

        1. Not universally accepted as illness or abnormality

        2. Even mental health professionals disagree

        3. Acceptance by general public still low

        4. Laws regarding homosexuality are being seriously reexamined—crime and punishment are being put aside

    H. Treatment of homosexuality

        1. May be appropriate if individual is unhappy, anxious, depressed, or dissatisfied with homosexuality

        2. Involves psychotherapy

II. Transsexuality

    A. The feeling that one belongs to the opposite sex

    B. Distinctively different from transvestism

C. Many transsexuals achieve happiness only after surgical and hormonal sex change procedures

III. Deviate Sexual Behavior

A. Concept of deviate sexuality depends on the context in which behavior occurs

B. Associated with mental illness and poor social adjustment

C. Certain deviate patterns can be discussed in terms of four types of psychopathology:

    1. Feelings of sexual insecurity

        a. Exhibitionism

        (1) The purposeful exposure of the penis to an unsuspecting female without intention of further sexual contact

        (2) Intention is usually to evoke fear and shock, not to solicit actual sexual contact

        (3) Exhibitionist is harmless, a nuisance rather than a danger

        b. Obscene phone calls

        (1) Caller desires shock reaction

        (2) Best way to handle call is to ignore caller and hang up

        c. Voyeurism

        (1) Voyeur attains sexual gratification by looking at sexual objects or situations

        (2) Most people have some degree of voyeuristic tendency

        (3) True "peeping Tom" usually feels shy and inferior and develops pattern of peeping plus masturbation; usually is harmless

    2. Mental incompetence

        a. Bestiality

        (1) Engaging in sexual contact with animals

        (2) Usually no important psychological motivations; animal is merely used as an aid in masturbation

        b. Incest

        (1) Sexual intercourse between individuals too closely related to marry legally

        (2) Most common among poor, unintelligent, or uneducated people

    3. Developmental abnormalities

        a. Pedophilia

        (1) Sexual involvement of an adult with a child

      (2) Either homosexual or heterosexual

      (3) Pedophiles usually suffer from arrested psychosexual development (fixation) or regression

   b. Fetishism

      (1) Sexual arousal from perception of inanimate objects

      (2) A degree of fetishism is normal

      (3) Heterosexual development is generally poor

   c. Transvestism

      (1) Wearing the clothing of the opposite sex

      (2) Transvestite may or may not be homosexual

 4. Disposition toward violent behavior

   a. Forcible rape

      (1) Rapist prefers rape to sex with willing partner

         (a) Entire way of life includes unnecessary violence

         (b) Rapist often hates women

         (c) Often a strong sadistic element in the rapist

      (2) To avoid rape, try to avoid high-risk situations

      (3) If rape seems unavoidable, better to cooperate—better to be raped and alive than raped and dead

   b. Sadism

      (1) The attainment of sexual satisfaction by inflicting cruelty on another person

      (2) Can take forms with no obvious sexual basis

   c. Masochism

      (1) The attainment of sexual gratification from suffering physical pain

      (2) Has been related to subconscious guilt feelings

Questions for Review

1. What are some of the common causes of homosexuality?

2. What is your own viewpoint on homosexuality?

3. Should a psychiatrist treat homosexuality as an emotional problem?

4. What is a lesbian?

5. Compare male and female patterns in homosexual relationships.

6. Contrast homosexuality, transvestism, and transsexuality.

7. What are the motivations of the typical rapist?

8. How are exhibitionism, voyeurism, and obscene calling related?

9. How do you distinguish an abnormal degree of fetishism?

10. What are some of the manifestations of sadism?

Chapter 5
FERTILITY

One of the most basic needs a baby carries with it into the world is a need for love and acceptance, the need to be wanted. An unwanted child often suffers lifelong emotional problems resulting from an unhappy childhood as the unloved and rejected product of an unplanned pregnancy. These emotional problems may be reflected in problems at school, delinquency and crime, and personal and social maladjustments. In addition, every unwanted child contributes to national and world population problems.

At the same time that children need to be wanted, adults need to be able to freely express their sexuality without fear of an unwanted pregnancy. It has been estimated (Connell, 1972) that in only about one in a thousand acts of sexual intercourse is pregnancy a desired goal. Thus the effective use of safe and adequate contraceptive methods is of obvious importance both to adults and to their children.

About Unwanted Pregnancies

Numerous studies have clearly shown that unwanted pregnancies among unmarried college students seldom result from a lack of knowledge, but from a lack of motivation to use birth control methods. This lack of motivation is closely related to internal conflict about accepting oneself as a sexual person or about the propriety of nonmarital intercourse. Most effective birth control methods require some advance planning—a prescription must be obtained and filled, or a product purchased. Such advance planning entails conscious and rational acceptance of the likelihood of sexual intercourse. For someone who cannot accept himself or herself as a sexual, adult person or who has strong conflicting emotions about nonmarital sexual intercourse, such conscious acceptance may be impossible. If sex just "happens" rather than being planned, the person can avoid the emotional discomfort or guilt involved in a conscious decision.

Selecting a Method

Methods of controlling birth fall into four general categories: sexual abstinence, contraception, sterilization, and abortion. Sexual abstinence is the avoidance of sexual intercourse either temporarily or permanently. Contraception is the interference, either by chemical or physical means, with ovulation, fertilization, or implantation of the fertilized egg. Sterilization is the surgical alteration of the reproductive system to eliminate the possibility of impregnation. Abortion is the surgical or chemical termination of a pregnancy before term. Each of these methods has its advantages and disadvantages.

In selecting the best method for a given situation, an important factor is *safety*. The ideal method would neither harm health nor reduce the capacity for future parenthood. It should be free from harmful or unwanted side effects, both for the person using the method and for the partner. A second factor is the *rate of effectiveness* (Table 5.1). It must be effective in prevent-

TABLE 5.1 Effectiveness of Fertility Control Methods

Method	Pregnancies per 100 Woman-Years	
	Theoretical Effectiveness[1]	Average Use-Effectiveness[2]
No contraception	80	80
Rhythm	15	40
Douche	?	30
Withdrawal	15	30
Spermicidal preparations	5	15–25
Diaphragm	5	15–25
Condom	5	15–25
Condom and spermicidal foam	1	5
IUD	1–3	3–10
Mini-pills	2–3	5
Sequential pills	1–2	3–5
Combination pills	0.1	1–2
Sterilization	near 0	near 0
Abortion	0	0

[1]Theoretical effectiveness is the maximum effectiveness of the method when used properly and consistently.
[2]Average use-effectiveness is the effectiveness of the method when used by large numbers of people over long periods of time.
Figures compiled from various sources.

ing pregnancy for the particular person. It should also have "use-effectiveness," or a high probability of continued use. The third factor is *ease of administration*. It is expected that any permanent device, like an intrauterine device (IUD), will be inserted by a professional. If a temporary device is used, the person must find it easy to apply. Ideally, the device will be one which is applied at some time other than during actual preparation for intercourse. A fourth element is *acceptability*. Acceptance must include factors such as medical (one's medical history, absence of side effects, physical comfort), social (prevailing religions, cultural hesitations), and psychological (personal aesthetics, one's own habits and attitudes). *Reversibility* is a fifth element. Sixth is *expense*. Some devices (such as the IUD) require only an initial expense, while others involve a recurring cost (pills, condom, foams). Even in the United States, economy is a factor for many couples, but in some countries several cents a day may be a prohibitive cost. Last is the effect the device has on sex drive and the pleasures of intercourse. It is natural to want the assurance that such feelings will not be reduced. A couple must be satisfied they have chosen the method of birth control that best suits their needs.

Withdrawal (Coitus Interruptus)

This method consists of withdrawing the penis from the vagina just before ejaculation. This is an ancient technique and is mentioned in the Old Testament scripture. It was a common method prior to the development of mechanical and chemical contraceptives and is still commonly used.

To be effective the man must be alert to the first signs of orgasm and be prepared to terminate intercourse at any moment. Even before ejaculation, the drops of clear fluid found on the end of the penis are carrying sperm (in fact, about 50,000 sperm per drop). If even these drops get into the vagina there may be good chance of pregnancy.

The disadvantages of this method are numerous. Its effectiveness is low. For every one hundred couples practicing this method for one year, thirty women are likely to become pregnant. Equally important, stopping intercourse just before orgasm greatly intereferes with enjoyment of intercourse for both people. On the positive side, it can be said that withdrawal requires no preparation, no medical supervision, and no expense. Yet for those wishing effective birth control, withdrawal is not a good choice.

The Rhythm Method

This method is based on the fact that fertilization is more likely if intercourse occurs one or two days before or after ovulation. The couple assumes that ovulation occurs about the middle of the menstrual cycle. The idea is that if they avoid intercourse during this time, they can prevent pregnancy. This all sounds good, assuming that ovulation does indeed occur at midmonth.

Ordinarily a woman produces a ripe egg about 14 days before the start of the next menstruation (Figure 5.1). Ovulation is tied more closely to the next onset of menstruation than to the last one. But even assuming that a woman has invariable menstrual periods 28 days apart (the mature egg actually may be released anywhere from the seventeenth to the thirteenth day before the next menstruation begins), there is little way of predicting in any given cycle exactly when ovulation will occur. To be safe, a woman must refrain from intercourse on these five days. Yet intercourse two days prior to earliest ovulation could still leave live sperm to fertilize the egg, and intercourse a day after the latest possible ovulation could mean an egg was still present to be fertilized. Just for insurance, it is recommended that the couple refrain from intercourse from the nineteenth to twelfth day before the woman's next menstrual discharge, or from Day 10 to Day 17 after the beginning of her last discharge. For a period of eight days each month, she must not have intercourse.

Most women, of course, do not menstruate with such clocklike regularity. Some women have menstrual cycles as short as 18 days, and others as long as several months. The average woman may vary as much as eight to nine days between her shortest and longest cycles. Some women, perhaps as many as 15 out of every 100, have menstrual cycles so irregular

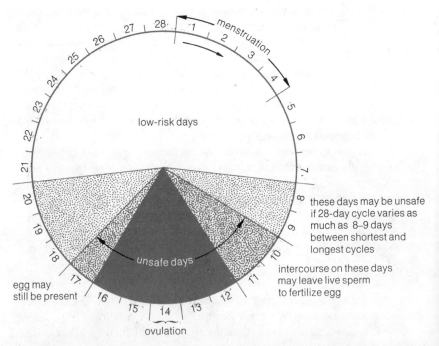

Figure 5.1 *Theory of the rhythm method. The shaded sections indicate days of greatest chance of pregnancy (the greater the shading, the greater the chance). This chart is based on an average 28-day menstrual cycle*

they cannot use the rhythm method at all. Following childbirth the cycles may be upset for several months and ovulation time may be unpredictable.

Regulating sex by the calendar rather than by the way a person feels does not appeal to many couples. Even faithful adherence is not highly effective in preventing pregnancy. Of 100 women practicing this method for a year, 40 can expect to become pregnant.

Mechanical Contraceptives

The Condom ("Rubber")

The condom is usually a synthetic rubber sheath (Figure 5.2) worn rather tightly over the erect penis and fitted with a rubber ring at the open end to help hold it in place. The function of the condom is to prevent the sperm from reaching the vagina. It is at least as effective as the diaphragm in preventing pregnancy, and its effectiveness can be increased if it is used in conjunction with a contraceptive jelly applied to the outside of the condom or foam inserted into the vagina before intercourse.

The condom is used widely around the world both for the prevention of venereal disease and the control of pregnancy. Its use also combats *Trichomonas* infection and reduces the chances of transmission of *Herpes* virus. It is sometimes useful to men bothered by premature ejaculation, since it reduces penile sensations. It is one of the handiest methods to use

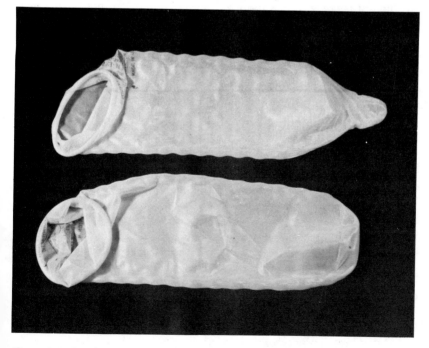

Figure 5.2 *Condoms. Above, plain end; below, receptacle end.*

and can be purchased almost anywhere for from 10 cents to $1.50 per condom. It has no side effects and is fully "reversible" once discontinued. Until the availability of the pill and the IUD, it was one of the more effective methods of birth control. Even today the use of a quality condom along with a contraceptive foam (by the woman) offers good protection.

There are drawbacks though. The condom interferes with the full enjoyment of intercourse by dulling the man's sensations, and it requires interruption of the act to put it in place. Condoms are subject to breakage, and they can come off during intercourse.

The failure rate of the condom can be reduced by taking several precautions. First, only high-quality condoms should be purchased. The U.S. Food and Drug Administration has found that as many as 5 percent of cheaper condoms have holes in them. Since condoms are made of very thin rubber, they should be handled with care. To avoid damage, the condom should be placed on the penis just prior to vaginal penetration.

The condom, like other contraceptives, should be used throughout the menstrual cycle, rather than just when the woman's fertility seems most likely. Otherwise a couple is, in effect, taking the same risk of pregnancy as if the rhythm system were used.

The penis should be withdrawn from the vagina promptly after ejaculation to prevent semen from working out over the top of the condom. Some condoms have a small saclike receptacle end which helps prevent this type of leakage, but withdrawal should still be prompt. Use a new condom for each intercourse.

The Diaphragm

The vaginal diaphragm, sold widely in the United States, is a shallow rubber or synthetic rubber cup designed to cover the cervix and thus prevent sperm from entering the uterus (Figure 5.3). Since the wrong size diaphragm may slip out of place or be displaced during intercourse, a woman must be fitted with a diaphragm by a physician. The woman then commonly purchases the diaphragm by prescription at a drug store. Since a woman's vagina is stretched by childbirth, her diaphragm should be checked for fit after delivery.

A contraceptive jelly or cream containing a *spermicide* (material that kills sperm on contact) should always be used with the diaphragm. Jelly should be applied around the edge and on both sides of the diaphragm prior to insertion. Masters and Johnson have shown that the vagina widens and elongates during sexual excitement (Figure 3.3) and that even the best fitting diaphragm moves quite freely in the vagina. Cream on the inner side of the diaphragm serves to protect the cervix from wandering sperm.

The diaphragm can be inserted two to four hours in advance and must be left in place for eight hours after intercourse.

A diaphragm properly fitted and inserted will not be felt by the woman and will not impair sexual sensation for either partner. It may be left in

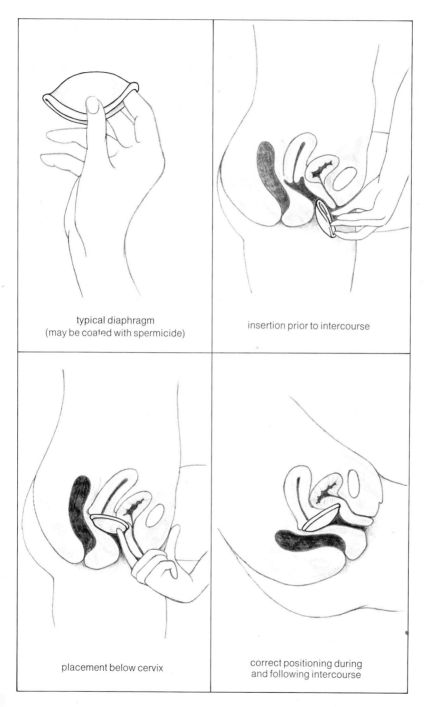

typical diaphragm
(may be coated with spermicide)

insertion prior to intercourse

placement below cervix

correct positioning during
and following intercourse

Figure 5.3   *The diaphragm*

position for 24 hours without any harm or discomfort to the woman. After removal, the diaphragm should be washed and dried; with such care it should last for several years.

The use of the diaphragm requires continuous, high motivation. While the diaphragm was once quite popular, today less than 10 percent of couples use this technique. Nor is its effectiveness too great. Out of 100 women using it for one full year, 15 to 25 are likely to become pregnant.

Intrauterine Device (IUD)

The IUD has been used for centuries. The devices vary in size, shape, and kind of material (Figure 5.4). The coil-like devices are preformed and may be inserted by being pushed through a small pencil-sized tube into the uterus where they resume their initial shape. Devices of other shapes may be applied with aid of anesthesia. The devices may be made of plastic, stainless steel, and recently some have appeared of plastic wrapped in copper.

Once in place, the device can often remain there without any harmful effects to the patient. No other contraceptive protection is necessary, and the woman wearing it should be totally unaware of its presence. The devices have a nylon thread attached which protrudes into the vagina. Prior to intercourse a woman should check the thread with her finger to be certain the device is still in place.

The IUD is completely "reversible." When the woman decides to become pregnant, the device is removed. Before long the uterus is again

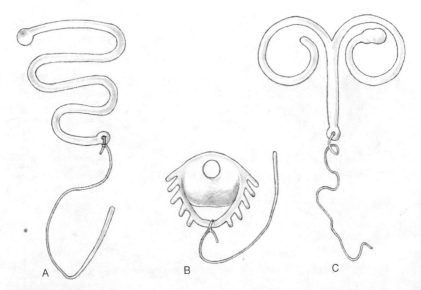

Figure 5.4 *Intrauterine devices commonly available: (A) Lippes loop, (B) Dalkon shield, (C) "Saf-T-Coil"*

functioning in a normal way, and within one month to a year most women become pregnant.

Older women and those with the greater number of children tend to tolerate and retain an IUD better than younger women and those with fewer children. Newer designs, however, are proving successful for child-less women. Bleeding and cramping are frequently corrected by changing to a smaller IUD.

Out of 100 women using the device for one year, about three to ten can expect to become pregnant. In the event a pregnancy takes place while the device is still in the uterus, the IUD does not interfere with the normal development of the unborn child or with its delivery. The use of the IUD is unrelated to sexual intercourse, requires no daily motivation, involves no cost beyond that of initial insertion, and has no effect whatsoever on a woman's hormone levels. There is great hope for worldwide use of the IUD today in terms of its low cost, ease of insertion, and long-term effectiveness.

Chemical Contraceptives

The Douche

Some women believe that pregnancy can be prevented by douching —washing the semen out of the vagina. Various douches have been used, such as hot water, cold water, vinegar, lemon juice, soap chips dissolved in water, or washes available in drug stores. A large rubber bulb, or syringe, is filled with the fluid and emptied into the vagina.

Of 100 women using the douche method for one year, about 30 are apt to become pregnant. The reason for the low effectiveness of douching is that sperm are safely within the uterus within 30 seconds after ejaculation. A douche can wash out the vagina but not the uterus. Following unpro-tected ejaculation, regardless of how soon the douching is done and what is used, it is too late. In addition, the necessity for postorgasmic douching deprives both the man and woman of a warm and tender time together. Douching cannot be considered to be a good contraceptive method.

Vaginal Spermicides

Various chemical preparations kill or impede the movement of sperm. These vaginal spermicides are available in the form of creams, jellies, aerosol foams, and suppositories.

Creams and jellies are usually used with a diaphragm, while the others, which tend to be somewhat stronger, are usually used without any other contraceptive device. The woman inserts a measured amount of the spermicide into the vagina with a special applicator one hour or less prior to each intercourse (Figure 5.5). The applicator deposits the preparation high in the vaginal tract at the opening into the uterus. One application is good for only one intercourse. The action of the preparations is twofold: the spermicide acts to kill the sperm on contact; the chemical base of the

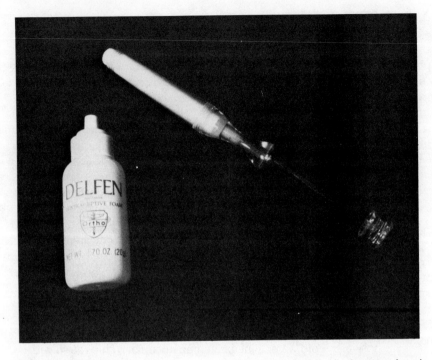

Figure 5.5   *Contraceptive foam. Using the plastic applicator, the foam is placed into the vagina over the cervix.*

preparation forms a coating that keeps surviving sperm from entering the uterus. The effectiveness of jellies alone in preventing pregnancy is not good. Out of 100 women using this method for one year, about 25 are apt to become pregnant.

Vaginal foam is a variation on the creams. It is packaged in a can under pressure or in individual measured dose dispensers. The foam contents are released into a plastic applicator, by which the foam is applied high in the vagina. Foams are effective in preventing pregnancy in all but about 15 women out of 100 per year.

Suppositories and foaming tablets are solid spermicides that melt or dissolve when placed in the vagina. A suppository is a small pencil-shaped glycerin-gelatin preparation containing a spermicide that melts at body temperature. It is inserted deep into the vagina from a few minutes to an hour before intercourse. Enough time must be allowed for it to melt before intercourse begins. Suppositories may be purchased without a prescription and are harmless. Their reliability in preventing pregnancy is about the same as the creams or jellies used alone.

Foaming tablets dissolve on contact with the moisture in the vagina. They release a gas that spreads the spermicide over the upper vaginal area. A tablet should be inserted several minutes to an hour before intercourse.

They can be purchased without prescription at drug stores. Their effectiveness in preventing pregnancy is considered to be less than creams or jellies used alone.

The action of the vaginal spermicides is completely reversible when discontinued. They do require use at some time relatively close to coitus and require memory and motivation on the part of the woman to insure effectiveness.

Hormonal Contraceptives

The female oral contraceptive pills (the Pill) are designed to prevent ovulation or implantation of the fertilized egg. These pills, which are highly effective in preventing pregnancy, are composed of female hormones. You will recall from our discussion in Chapter 2 that the pituitary gland produces the hormones FSH and LH, which are necessary for the production and release of a mature egg in the ovary. The follicles in the ovary produce both estrogen and progesterone. Among other functions, the estrogen inhibits the production of FSH and progesterone inhibits the production of LH. When the pill is taken daily, starting with Day 5 after the beginning of menstruation, the presence of progestin (synthetic progesterone) and estrogen inhibit the body's production of FSH and LH before a mature egg is produced. Ovulation does not occur and no egg is present to unite with the sperm released during intercourse. The woman thus fails to become pregnant. This suppression of egg production is very much like the suppression of egg production that takes place while a woman is pregnant. Under the influence of natural estrogen and progesterone, no other mature eggs are produced until after the pregnancy has terminated.

Various types of pills are produced today, including the combined pills, the sequential pills, the mini-pills and the morning-after pills.

The Combined Pills

The original pills combined estrogen and progestin. Most combined pills are designed to be taken for 20 or 21 days of the menstrual cycle, starting on Day 5 and ending on Day 24 or 25. Then for seven or eight days the pill is omitted, allowing menstruation to occur. Some women experience side effects such as nausea, headache, swelling of the breasts, and bleeding. Commonly these symptoms diminish or disappear after the first several months. In addition to preventing ovulation, the combined pill also makes the uterine lining less receptive to a fertilized egg, thus adding to the pill's effectiveness. Of 1000 women using the combined pill properly for one year, only one is apt to become pregnant (0.1 pregnancy per 100 women for one year).

The Sequential Pills

Because of complaints about the side effects of the combined pill, the sequential pills were developed. They amount to two different pills, one taken from Day 5 through Day 19 and the other from Day 20 through Day 24. (The days differ for different brands.) The pills taken the first 15 days contain estrogen only; the pills taken the last 5 days contain both estrogen and progestin (like the combined pill). The sequential pills are packaged so that the pills are easily taken in the right order. The action of both pills is similar. The sequential pill is less effective than the combined pill. Of 100 women taking the sequential pill for one year, three to five are apt to become pregnant. Depending on the brand used, there are minor variations in the dosage and number of pills taken. There are 20-, 21-, or 28-pill packages. The latter utilize placebo tablets for 7 out of 28 days, which have no chemical effect but keep the woman in the habit of taking the pill every day.

The major advantage of all pill methods is their effectiveness and simplicity. The pill is taken at a time other than during sexual intercourse. Obviously, for the method to work, the woman must be motivated to take the pill and remember to do so. When a woman wants to become pregnant, she merely stops taking the pill, and she should become pregnant with at least the same likelihood as before taking the pill.

Mini-Pills

The so-called mini-pills contain small doses of synthetic progesterone. Unlike other oral contraceptives, they are taken daily without interruption rather than cyclically. Also unlike other oral contraceptives, they do not act to prevent ovulation. Rather, they prevent fertilization by thickening the mucus plug in the cervix or prevent implantation by altering the uterine lining. Mini-pills are less reliable than other types of oral contraceptives, with a pregnancy rate of about 5 per 100 woman-years. However, they have the advantage of causing far fewer side effects than combined or sequential pills.

The Morning-After Pill

A woman may find herself in a situation where she engages in sexual intercourse without having access to a birth control device. Faced with the very real possibility of pregnancy, the morning-after pill may be used to insure against pregnancy after she has had intercourse. It takes several days for a fertilized egg to move to the uterus and several more for it to implant in the uterine lining. A series of morning-after pills taken three to five days after intercourse may prevent implantation. Consisting of large doses of stilbesterol, a synthetic estrogen, the pill causes contraction of the uterus and the expulsion of its contents. Not to be used as a regular birth control method, it was meant to be effectively used on an emergency basis. It often causes temporary nausea and is known to cause cancers. If the morning-after pill fails to prevent pregnancy, abortion should be considered.

On the Safety of Pills

There has been much controversy about the safety of the oral contraceptives. Like so many other decisions in life, the decision of whether or not to take pills involves weighing the relative hazards of each course of action. The pill involves risk; pregnancy also involves risk.

One concern is cancer. While there is no evidence that the pill causes cancer, it is known to accelerate the growth of existing cancers of the female organs (such as the uterus or breast). Thus most physicians require a routine Pap smear to detect uterine cancer and a breast examination every six months for all women taking the pill. As a result, there are actually *fewer* cancer deaths among women on the pill, as most of their cancers are detected in an early, curable stage.

Another concern is the formation of blood clots in the veins. Women (especially of blood type A) do run a four- to seven-fold increased risk of such clots when taking the pill but an even higher risk when pregnant.

Also, after several years on pills, some women develop abnormalities in their blood-sugar levels. These problems seem to reverse themselves if the pills are discontinued. In addition, there are many other low-incidence problems which may or may not be associated with the pill.

In sum, the pills are fundamentally safe, but they can cause trouble for some women. It is most important that the pills be taken only under a physician's supervision and that they be discontinued if any serious problem develops.

Experimental Contraceptives

Other hormonal contraceptives are now under investigation. The "20-year pill" is implanted under the skin and gradually releases its contents. A woman wanting a child would have her physician remove the pill. Pills for men are being investigated that would make conception impossible by preventing the development of sperm or making sperm incapable of uniting with the egg. Vaccination appears to be another possibility. This would involve making the woman immune to sperm by injecting her with antibodies that would attack and reject sperm.

Sterilization

Sterilization is a permanent method of fertility control that is virtually 100 percent effective. A man or woman who has been properly sterilized can have children only if a second operation is successfully performed to undo the work of the first. Sterilization does not remove any of the sex organs or glands and has no effect upon sexual desire or performance.

For a woman, the operation, called a *tubal ligation*, consists of cutting the two Fallopian tubes and closing off the cut ends (Figure 5.6). It can be done as part of a cesarean delivery, by abdominal incision, by a laparo-

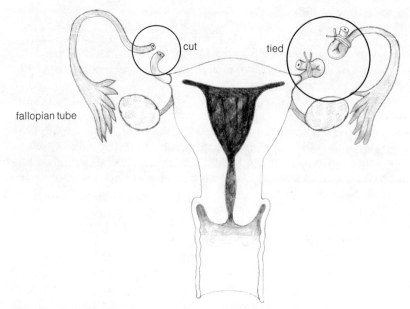

cut   tied

fallopian tube

Figure 5.6   *Tubal ligation, or sterilization by severing the fallopian tubes*

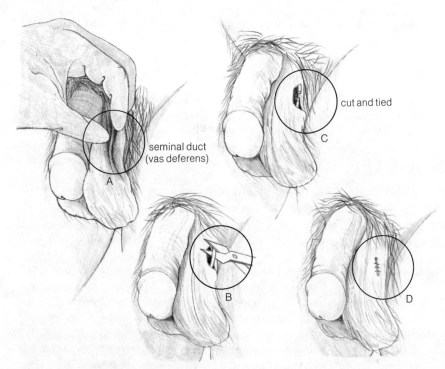

seminal duct
(vas deferens)

cut and tied

A

B

C

D

Figure 5.7   *Vasectomy, or sterilization by severing the vas deferens*

scope, or by way of the vagina. Once the tubes have been tied, the sperm can no longer reach the egg, and the egg can no longer reach the uterus.

For a man, the operation, called a *vasectomy*, consists of cutting and tying the vas deferens, the passages through which sperm travel from the testes to the genital passages (Figure 5.7). It requires only small cuts on both sides of the scrotum and can be safely performed in a physician's office. Following vasectomy, mature sperm may remain in the passages for up to six weeks. Contraceptives should be used for sexual intercourse until a sperm count confirms the absence of sperm in the semen. The man continues to produce seminal fluid as before; it is still ejaculated upon orgasm, but it contains no sperm. The sperm disintegrate and are absorbed by blood vessels in the testes.

Once a sterilization is performed, no daily motivation or remembering is required to prevent pregnancy. The main problem is its low rate of "reversibility." Only 35 to 50 percent of sterilized people can be restored to fertility.

Sterilization is legally permissible in every state of the union, as well as in many countries throughout the world. A few states require a medical reason for the operation.

Therapeutic Abortion

In 1973, the United States Supreme Court ruled that therapeutic abortion should be freely available, within certain guidelines, to any woman in the United States. This ruling took precedence over laws that still prohibited abortion in many states and thus made abortion legal in the whole country. About the only restrictions remaining on abortion are those requiring that the procedure be performed by a licensed physician and that it occur before the fetus can survive on its own outside the uterus. This ruling does not mean that the controversy over abortion is over. Anti-abortion forces are still campaigning vigorously for a return to more restrictive abortion laws.

As it now stands, any woman, regardless of her motivation, may have an early pregnancy terminated legally by a qualified physician under sanitary conditions. Under such conditions, abortion is extremely safe —much safer, in fact, than a full-term pregnancy and delivery. There is absolutely no reason to resort to self-abortion or abortion by other than a qualified physician, both of which entail considerable risk of infection, hemorrhage, or other complications.

Despite abortion's legality, it is not the ideal solution to unwanted pregnancy for women whose religious backgrounds or other values cause them to seriously doubt the morality of abortion. Such women should consider other ways of dealing with their pregnancy so that they can avoid the guilt or regret brought on by consenting to an abortion. It should be emphasized, however, that among women in general, the incidence of emotional conflicts following abortion is quite low.

There are several commonly used methods of aborting pregnancies. A *dilatation and curettage* ("D and C") is a dilating of the cervix and a mild scraping of the inside of the uterus. This method may be safe up through the twelfth week of pregnancy. With the *suction curettage* (suction aspiration) negative pressure is used to suck out the contents of the uterus. It may be safely used up through the twelfth week, or in conjunction with a "D and C," up through the seventeenth week. Another method is to introduce a *hypertonic solution* of saline or glucose into the uterine cavity. The uterus starts to contract and, within about 24 to 48 hours, the fetus and placenta should be expelled. It may be used up to 24 weeks of pregnancy. This method can be difficult and must be performed only by a qualified physician. If improperly administered it may result in serious infection or death to the woman. A physician may also resort to *abdominal surgery* to either remove the fetus from the uterus by cesarean-like section (hysterotomy) or to remove the uterus (hysterectomy). This may be used for pregnancies up through 24 weeks. All of the above methods are safe only when handled by a qualified physician.

Some controversy surrounds the procedure called *menstrual extraction*, or *menstrual regulation*. In this simple procedure, a period delayed for any reason for five to ten days is extracted from the uterus by a small tube inserted through the cervix and connected to a vacuum device. No attempt is made to determine whether the woman is pregnant. Thus menstrual extraction may or may not constitute abortion. The controversy centers around who performs the procedure (it is often performed by volunteers in so-called women's clinics or even by women upon themselves), its safety (which probably depends upon who performs it), and its possible widespread adoption as a replacement for contraception.

Regardless of the type of abortion, few people would argue that it should take the place of contraception. Many people feel, however, that abortion must be readily available as a back-up method of fertility control for those who find themselves with an unwanted pregnancy.

Infertility

Some couples who practice no form of birth control would like to have children but have none at all. Other couples wish for more children than they have but are unable to have more. Out of every 100 married couples, 10 are unable to have children and 15 have fewer than they would like. This means that about 25 percent of the population is troubled with insufficient fertility.

There are actually two levels of insufficient fertility. Only the temporary inability to produce children is termed *infertility*. A total inability to produce them is called *sterility*.

Causes of Infertility

Infertility may be due to physical defects, emotional stress, a mistiming of ovulation, or a sperm allergy. Either partner or both may be the source of the problem. For every 100 cases of infertility, the woman is unable to conceive in 50 to 55 percent of the cases, the man in 30 to 35 percent of them, and the problem is shared by both partners in about 15 percent of cases.

MALE INFERTILITY

In the male the problem is a failure to ejaculate enough active sperm to reach and fertilize the egg. This difficulty has no relation to the man's masculinity, since the male hormones and the sperm are produced by different cells. A man may be sterile and still be sexually normal in all other respects.

Failure in sperm production may be due to illnesses (mumps or other diseases), occupational hazards (exposure to X rays, radioactive substances, certain metals or chemicals, gasoline fumes and carbon monoxide, or excessive heat), sedentary living, obesity, tight under-clothing, infrequent coitus, habits (excessive smoking or drinking), poor health, inadequate nutrition, or emotional stress. Other causes for male infertility can be blockage of the ducts (from birth defect or infection) or varicocele (a swelling of the veins on the vas deferens). These conditions may often be corrected surgically.

Techniques have been devised to improve the concentration of sperm. The first drops of semen contain a far greater number of sperm than the later discharge. In some cases a man is advised to withdraw the penis after the first portions of ejaculated sperm have entered the vagina to prevent dilution of the first drops. Some physicians have collected first semen drops from several ejaculations, combined them, and introduced them artificially into the uterus of the woman.

FEMALE INFERTILITY

The female reproductive system is not only more complicated than the male; it must also respond to the interaction of some critical hormones. Thus the causes for infertility in the woman can be more complex.

The first fact that must be known is whether a mature egg, which can be fertilized, is available each month. In order to determine whether ovulation is occurring, the physician may take basal body temperature readings (BBT's) or remove and examine tissue from the uterus that should show changes in the event of ovulation. Depending on the cause, failure to ovulate (by far the most common cause of infertility in women) may be treated surgically, hormonally, or by medication. Some women begin ovulating after taking an oral contraceptive for several months and then stopping.

Infertility can also be due to abnormal functioning of the genital system, abnormal genetic development of ova, undersecretion of gonado-tropic hormones, salpingitis (inflammation and fibrous formation within the Fallopian tubes), or vaginal fluids that kill the sperm. The egg may be fertilized properly, but unable to attach to the uterine wall. This may be due to hormonal imbalance that alters the nature of the uterine lining.

There is also some evidence that secretions from the vagina and/or cervix in some women may inactivate sperm. In these women, the chances for conception appear to improve if the woman is removed from contact with sperm for a period of time through either abstinence or by use of a condom. It is believed that there may be an antisperm activity in some women, perhaps the production of an antibody or antibody-like substance. If so, the man's use of a condom can avert the sperm contact with the woman, yet allow for frequent intercourse.

TIMING OF INTERCOURSE

To achieve pregnancy, it is important that intercourse occur near the time of ovulation. In ruling out possible mistiming of intercourse as a cause for infertility, it is recommended that the woman keep records of her body temperature in an attempt to determine the time of egg release. In order to save up sperm, some physicians recommend that an infertile couple refrain from intercourse during the days just before the fertile period, and then repeat intercourse at 48-hour intervals during the fertile period.

Overcoming Infertility

A couple ought to consult their family physician if they are not able to conceive after several months. In the event a family physician feels his training is insufficient for the problem or is unable to find the cause, he may refer the patient or couple to a specialist or clinic. Medical schools often have fertility clinics. Help may also be obtained from a local Planned Parenthood Committee. If the couple does not know where to find such a clinic, they may write to: Planned Parenthood, 515 Madison Avenue, New York, New York 10022, for referral information. Another source is the American Fertility Society, 944 S. 18th Street, Birmingham, Alabama 35205.

Artificial Insemination

In the discussion of male infertility, we referred to placing semen into the uterus by means other than sexual intercourse. *Artificial insemination*, or therapeutic insemination, as some prefer to call it, involves the use of the husband's semen or that from another donor. The semen is introduced into the woman by one of several mechanical means of the physician's choosing. More commonly, the semen is donated by a nonhusband due to the husband's inability to produce either sufficient sperm or sufficient normal sperm.

Adoption

Some couples who want children are never able to have them. They may satisfy their desire for a family by adopting children.

Adoption is a common practice today. There are, in fact, more couples desiring adopted children than there are children to be placed. In certain localities, qualified couples often wait years to receive an adopted child.

Summary

I. About Unwanted Pregnancies

    A. Result from lack of use of birth control, not lack of knowledge of methods

    B. Most common cause of failure to use birth control is internal conflict about sexuality or nonmarital sex

    C. Allowing sex to just "happen" avoids emotional discomfort or guilt

    D. Effective birth control requires advance planning

II. Selecting a Method—Considerations Include

    A. Safety

    B. Effectiveness

    C. Effect on future fertility

    D. Cost

    E. Effect on enjoyment of sex

    F. Acceptability

III. Withdrawal (Coitus Interruptus)

    A. Withdrawal of penis from vagina prior to ejaculation

    B. An ancient method; still commonly used

    C. Many disadvantages:

        1. Not highly effective (30 pregnancies per 100 woman-years)

        2. Interferes with sexual pleasure

IV. The Rhythm Method

    A. An attempt to avoid intercourse during fertile period of each menstrual cycle

    B. Not highly effective (40 pregnancies per 100 woman-years)

    C. Ovulation is too unpredictable for success

V. The Condom (Rubber)

    A. Thin sheath worn over erect penis during intercourse

   B. Prevents semen from entering vagina

   C. Fairly reliable; highly reliable if used with contraceptive foam or jelly

   D. Also helps prevent VD transmission

   E. Readily available

   F. Some dulling of sensation of intercourse

   G. For maximum effectiveness:

      1. Purchase reliable brand, preferably with receptacle end

      2. Handle carefully

      3. Use at all times

      4. Withdraw penis from vagina promptly after ejaculation

      5. Do not reuse

VI. The Diaphragm

   A. Shallow rubber cup worn in vagina to prevent sperm from entering uterus

   B. Size must be prescribed by physician

   C. Used with contraceptive jelly around edge

   D. Must be left in place for eight hours after intercourse

   E. Successful use requires high motivation

   F. Pregnancy rate of 15 to 25 per 100 woman-years

VII. Intrauterine Device (IUD)

   A. Device inserted into uterus to prevent pregnancy

   B. Various sizes, shapes, materials

   C. Inserted by physician, left in place until pregnancy is desired

   D. Low incidence of serious side effects

   E. Many advantages:

      1. Completely reversible when pregnancy desired

      2. Effectiveness—3 to 10 pregnancies per 100 woman-years

      3. Use is unrelated to sexual intercourse

      4. After insertion, requires no additional expense or motivation

VIII. Chemical Contraceptives

   A. The douche

      1. An attempt to wash semen from the vagina before sperm enter the uterus

      2. Not effective—about 30 pregnancies per 100 woman-years

B. Vaginal spermicides

1. Various foams, creams, jellies, and suppositories containing sperm-killing chemicals

2. Used alone, foam more effective than other products

a. Foam—about 15 pregnancies per 100 woman-years

b. Others—about 25 pregnancies per 100 woman-years

IX. Hormonal Contraceptives

A. Oral contraceptives (the Pill) act to prevent ovulation or implantation

1. Contain estrogen and/or synthetic progesterone

2. Suppress production of FSH and LH by pituitary

B. Combined pills

1. Contain both estrogen and progestin

2. Taken for 20 or 21 days each menstrual cycle, starting on day 5

3. Properly used, allow only 1 pregnancy per 1000 woman-years

C. Sequential pills

1. Two types pills in each cycle:

a. First 15 contain estrogen only

b. Last 5 contain estrogen and progestin

2. Lower incidence of minor side effects than combined pills (same incidence of major side effects)

3. Less reliable than combined pills—3 to 5 pregnancies per 100 woman-years

D. Mini-pills

1. Contain synthetic progesterone only

2. Taken daily, rather than cyclically

3. Prevent fertilization or implantation, rather than ovulation

4. Pregnancy rate about 5 per 100 woman-years

E. The Morning-After Pill

1. Taken within three to five days after intercourse, may prevent implantation of fertilized egg

2. Contains large doses of synthetic estrogen

3. Not for routine birth control

4. Often causes temporary nausea

     5. May cause cancer

     6. If pregnancy persists, abortion should be considered

  F. On safety of pills

     1. No evidence that pills cause cancer

     2. Do increase incidence of blood clots in veins

     3. In some women, may relate to blood-sugar level problems

     4. Risk of death from pills much lower than risk of death from pregnancy

     5. Should be taken only under physician's supervision

  G. Experimental contraceptives—many under investigation

X. Sterilization

  A. Should be considered permanent—low rate of reversibility

  B. Virtually 100 percent effective

  C. No effect on sexual desire or performance

  D. Female sterilization

     1. Tubal ligation—Fallopian tubes cut and tied off

     2. Various other techniques with same effect

  E. Male sterilization

     1. Vasectomy—vas deferens cut and tied off

     2. Done through small cuts on scrotum

     3. Seminal fluid still ejaculated, but contains no sperm

XI. Experimental contraceptives—many under investigation

XII. Therapeutic Abortion

  A. Made freely available to any woman in U.S. by 1973 Supreme Court decision

  B. Anti-abortion forces still campaigning for return to more restrictive abortion laws

  C. Methods include

     1. Dilatation and curettage (D and C)—scraping of inside of uterus

     2. Suction aspiration—removal of products of conception with mild vacuum

     3. Hypertonic solution—used later in pregnancy, injected into amniotic fluid, causes uterine contractions

     4. Surgical procedures

  D. Above methods safe only when performed by qualified physician

E. Menstrual extraction or menstrual regulation

    1. Delayed period extracted from uterus through small tube connected to vacuum device.

    2. Pregnancy not determined—may or may not constitute abortion.

    3. Often performed by volunteers in women's clinics.

    4. Still controversial.

XIII. Infertility—about 25 percent of couples troubled by insufficient fertility.

    A. Caused by either or both partners:

        1. Female—50 to 55 percent of cases.

        2. Male—30 to 35 percent of cases.

        3. Shared—about 15 percent of cases.

    B. Male

        1. Problem is failure to ejaculate sufficient, normal sperm.

        2. Causes include:

            a. Illness

            b. Occupational hazards

            c. Sedentary living

            d. Obesity

            e. Tight underclothing

            f. Infrequent coitus

            g. Excessive smoking or drinking

            h. Poor health

            i. Poor diet

            j. Emotional stress

            k. Blockage of sperm ducts

    C. Female

        1. As female reproductive system is more complicated, causes are likely to be complex and hard to find.

        2. Causes include:

            a. failure to ovulate.

            b. Oviducts unable to carry egg to uterus

            c. Uterine lining unfavorable for implantation

            d. vaginal secretions hostile to sperm.

D. Timing of intercourse—must be near ovulation for conception to occur.

E. Overcoming infertility

1. Couple should consult physician if unable to conceive after several months

2. Some physicians and clinics specialize in infertility

3. Artificial insemination—injection of semen directly into uterus by mechanical means

4. Adoption—desirable for many couples, but babies are in short supply

Questions for Review

1. What are some of the causes of unwanted pregnancies among people with adequate knowledge of contraceptive methods?

2. Is there a single best method of birth control? Explain.

3. Why is the rhythm method a generally unsatisfactory method of birth control?

4. What steps insure the maximum contraceptive effectiveness of the condom?

5. What are some advantages of an IUD?

6. Why is douching ineffective as birth control?

7. How do the conventional types of birth control pills work?

8. Who should consider sterilization as a fertility control method?

9. Just what is done in male and female sterilization? What effects do these procedures have on sexual intercourse?

10. What is menstrual extraction?

11. Compare the terms infertility and sterility.

12. What are some common causes of male infertility?

13. What are some causes of infertility in the female?

14. What is artificial insemination?

Chapter 6
PREGNANCY

In this section we will consider the course of a pregnancy from fertilization to delivery, with emphasis on the development of a healthy baby.

Fertilization

The human egg is viable (capable of living) only if it is fertilized within a day or two of ovulation. Since the movement of the egg through the oviduct (fallopian tube) from the ovary to the uterus requires three or four days, fertilization usually takes place somewhere in the upper portion of the oviduct. While only one sperm actually fertilizes the egg, it can penetrate the egg only when many other sperm cells surround the ovum. These attendant sperm cells give off enzymes that dissolve the tough exterior covering of the egg (Figures 6.1 and 6.2).

As soon as one sperm has penetrated the egg, the membrane covering the egg thickens and prevents the entry of other sperm. The nucleus in the head of the sperm then fuses with the nucleus in the egg, and fertilization has occurred.

The fertilized egg is now called a *zygote*. The zygote immediately begins to divide to form two cells, four cells, eight cells, and so on (Figure 6.3). It is now called an *embryo*.

Implantation

All the while this development is taking place, the embryo is being carried down the oviduct toward the uterus. The embryo spends about three days within the oviduct. By the time it leaves the oviduct and enters the uterus,

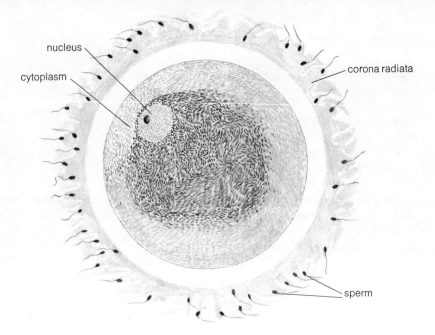

Figure 6.1 *Human ovum (egg)*

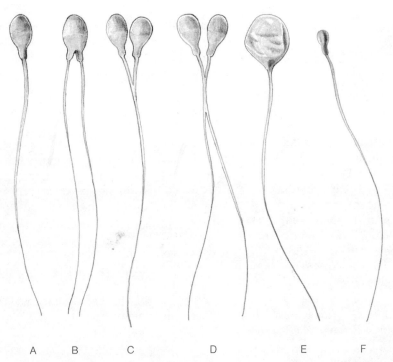

A   B   C   D   E   F

Figure 6.2 *Various forms of human sperm: (A) normal sperm, (B)–(F) abnormal sperm. Reduced fertility will result if the percentage of abnormal sperm reaches 25 percent of total sperm*

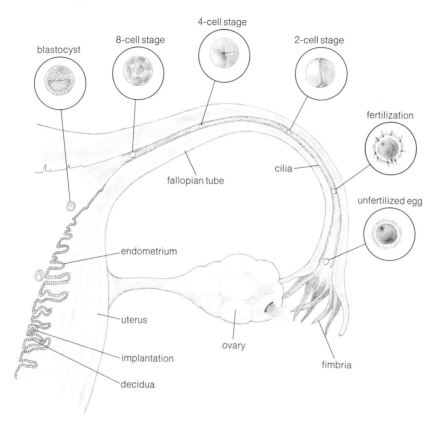

Figure 6.3 *Stages of development of zygote. The egg escapes from the follicle in the ovary, is picked up by the fallopian tube, and is fertilized by a sperm cell. It is moved through the tube into the uterus, and implants (buries) into the endometrium 6-8 days after fertilization. During this time the zygote divides into 2 cells, then 4, 8, and finally into a hollow ball of cells called a blastocyst*

the mass of cells looks like a hollow ball, but is actually filled with fluid. Even though the cell mass consists of many cells by this time, the whole mass is no larger than the undivided zygote.

For the next two or three days the embryo floats around in the cavity of the uterus. Then, at a site chosen by chance, the embryo attaches onto the lining of the uterus and begins to "take root." The site of this attachment, or *implantation*, is usually somewhere in the upper half of the uterus. The embryo sinks into the lining, which closes over it. Hence the embryo begins to increase in size, soon bulging into the cavity of the uterus, still completely surrounded with living tissue, now called *decidua*.

From the outer wall of the embryo, small fingerlike growths called *chorionic villi* begin to project into the decidua. In the decidua between the embryo and the uterine wall, spaces filled with maternal blood form (Figure 6.4). This area is known as the *placenta*. It serves to transfer

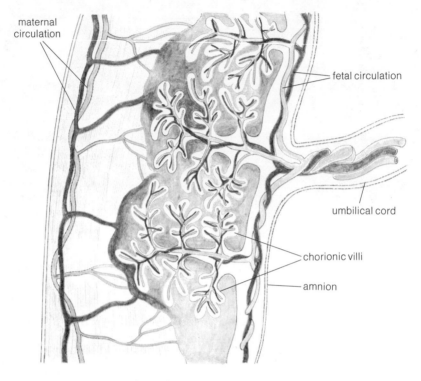

Figure 6.4   *A portion of the placenta*

nutrients from the mother to the child and wastes from the child to the mother. Even though there is a very close relation between the villi of the embryo and the tissues of the mother in the placenta, the two circulations are not directly connected. Blood does not cross from the mother to the embryo, and vice versa. The placenta actively transfers materials from the end of the fourth week after fertilization.

Amniotic Fluid

The embryo is attached to the placenta by the *umbilical cord*. It is surrounded by a double membrane consisting of the *amnion* and *chorion*. The space inside of these layers is often called the "bag of waters." The space is filled with *amniotic fluid*, which bathes the developing embryo (Figure 6.5). This fluid contains embryonic wastes which are exchanged with the mother's fluids. It also serves to give the embryo space in which to develop, protects it against injury, and keeps it at a constant temperature. Suspended and protected in a world of fluid and nourished through the placenta, the embryo develops with remarkable speed. By the eighth week, the embryo has taken on a distinctly human form, and it is known subsequently as the *fetus*.

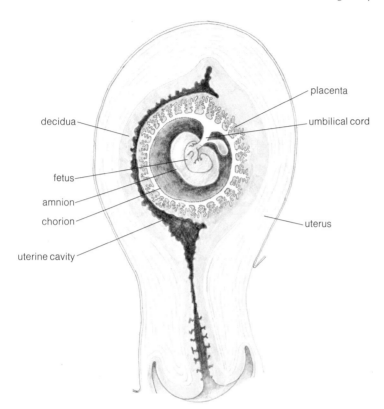

Figure 6.5 *Early fetal development*

Amniocentesis

The amniotic fluid contains chemical products released by the fetus as well as free-floating fetal cells. Thus examination of the amniotic fluid can reveal important information about the status of the embryo. In the diagnostic procedure known as *amniocentesis*, a sample of amniotic fluid is withdrawn from the uterine cavity through a hollow needle penetrating the abdominal and uterine walls (Figure 6.6). Chromosomal study of the embryonic cells and biochemical analysis of the fluid can reveal both the sex of the embryo and the presence or absence of any one of more than forty genetic disorders. Amniocentesis may be performed whenever the embryo is suspected of being genetically defective. It is highly recommended in cases where the woman has already given birth to a child suffering from Down's syndrome (mongolism) or certain other genetic disorders.

Determination of Sex

The cell's genetic information is contained in the chromosomes carried in the nucleus. Every normal human body cell contains 46 chromosomes. Of

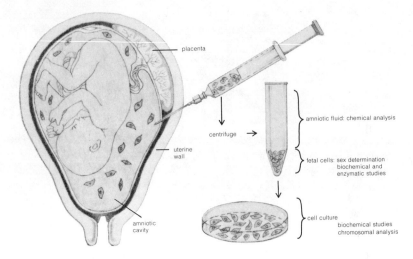

Figure 6.6 *Amniocentesis. A sample of amniotic fluid is withdrawn through a sterile needle, centrifuged, and checked for fetal defects as well as for the sex of the fetus.*

these, two are the *sex chromosomes*. There are two distinctive types of sex chromosomes: X and Y. In a normal female, each cell contains two X chromosomes; in a normal male, each cell contains one X and one Y. During the production of sperm and eggs, the number of chromosomes is halved. As a result, all normal human eggs contain one X chromosome. Half of all sperm contain an X chromosome, while the other half contain a Y. Thus the sex of the child is determined entirely by which type of sperm happens to fertilize the egg. An X-bearing sperm produces a daughter, while a Y-bearing sperm produces a son.

A Typical Pregnancy

A full-term pregnancy usually lasts about 266 days from conception, or until about 280 days after the beginning of the last menstrual period. This represents about nine calendar months.

A customary way of estimating the expected day of delivery is to count back three months from the first day of the last menstrual period and add seven days (Naegele's rule). For example, if a woman's last menstrual period began on June 10, the expected day of delivery would be March 17. Few mothers deliver on the expected day, and they may commonly deviate one to two weeks earlier or later than the expected date.

Diagnosis of Pregnancy

The first indication of pregnancy is often a missed menstrual period. One missed period is questionable evidence, but the second missed period strongly indicates pregnancy. The breasts may increase in size, firmness, and sensitivity. The nipples may become larger and darker. Nausea and vomiting ("morning sickness") are often associated with early pregnancy. Pressure of the uterus on the bladder may make urination more frequent.

A woman suspecting pregnancy should see a physician no later than the second missed period. The physician will examine the size and shape of the uterus and the condition of the cervix and probably administer a pregnancy test. A variety of pregnancy tests are in use, but most detect the presence of a specific hormone, *chorionic gonadotropin*, secreted by the chorion of the developing embryo and found in the blood and urine of a pregnant woman. Some of the newer tests are fairly reliable even in the first three or four weeks of pregnancy.

The most accurate signs of pregnancy directly concern the fetus. They include the detection of fetal heartbeat, perception of active movements of the fetus, and the ability to see the fetal skeleton in X-ray.

Prenatal Care

The care of the pregnant woman and her unborn baby is called prenatal care. While complications of pregnancy and delivery were once a major cause of death among women, modern prenatal care has reduced the hazards in pregnancy to a very low level. But the woman who fails to take advantage of prenatal care still exposes both herself and her baby to a high degree of danger. And, unfortunately, many women do not receive adequate prenatal care. This is especially true of lower-income women. It has been estimated, for instance, that one-third to one-half of the women delivering babies in tax-supported hospitals in large cities see a physician for the first time in their pregnancies only when they have already begun labor.

Since pregnancy makes great physical demands on the body, a disease or disorder that might normally have little effect on the woman can turn into a major complication when she is pregnant. Likewise, a condition only slightly affecting the mother can have a serious effect on the fetus. Careful medical supervision during pregnancy can avert many damaging conditions.

When a woman suspects that she is pregnant, she should have a complete physical examination, including blood tests and pelvic examination. Follow-up examinations should be made every four weeks until the seventh calendar month of pregnancy; then every two weeks, or more frequently as indicated, until the final month; then once a week until labor begins.

Morning Sickness

About 85 percent of all pregnant women experience a feeling of nausea (morning sickness) during the first three months of pregnancy. Experienced upon arising in the morning, it may be accompanied by vomiting.

If the vomiting does not disappear during the day, it is known as *pernicious vomiting*. It may become severe enough to interfere with nutrition, leading to dehydration and starvation. A physician can normally control this condition by the use of prescribed foods and drugs.

Diseases in Pregnancy

Many diseases assume an increased importance in pregnancy. During the early months of pregnancy, when the fetus is most vulnerable, the woman should try to avoid exposure to contagious diseases of any kind. Viruses are particularly damaging to the fetus. One of the most serious of these is rubella (German measles). German measles in the first six months of pregnancy may cause congenital disorders such as cataract, deafness, heart defects, or mental retardation. It is also thought to cause the death of the fetus in about one-fifth of cases where the mother contracts the disease early in pregnancy. Some states now require evidence of immunity to rubella (acquired through immunization or the actual disease) prior to issuing a marriage license.

Among bacterial diseases, syphilis and gonorrhea may create serious conditions. The spirochetes of syphilis will be transmitted from the mother to the fetus during the last half of pregnancy unless an infected mother receives treatment. Untreated syphilis frequently causes fetal damage or death. Gonorrhea during pregnancy may lead to infection of the eyes of the infant during delivery. A germicide is dropped into a child's eyes immediately after childbirth to prevent this infection.

Toxemias

Toxemias are a group of body poisonings that may occur during the last three months of pregnancy. They can cause serious complications, even death, to both the mother and the fetus. The conditions are all characterized by: a swelling of the body, particularly the feet or ankles; increased blood pressure; albumin in the urine (albuminuria); and a more-than-normal increase in body weight. Treatment by a physician may include a low-salt diet, complete bed rest, drugs to relax the mother and to reduce swelling, and prescribed amounts of water.

Diet in Pregnancy

The diet of the pregnant woman will have lifelong implications for her baby. Proper nutrition is important in the development of the fetal brain, bones, teeth, and other tissues. The diet must contain increased amounts of proteins, vitamins, and minerals. While physicians usually prescribe special vitamin preparations during pregnancy, an adequate intake of proteins and minerals normally depends on the mother's diet.

In recent years, many physicians have relaxed their restrictions on how much weight the pregnant woman should be allowed to gain. There is evidence that the birth weight of an infant is strongly associated with and conditioned by the weight gain of the mother, and that restriction of diet during pregnancy may unfavorably affect the growth and development of the fetus. The higher the infant's birth weight, the better his growth and performance during the first year of life. The Committee on Maternal Nutrition of the National Research Council is now recommending an average weight gain of 24 pounds (or a range from 20 to 25 pounds). This is particularly important for the low-weight woman whose weight before pregnancy is under 120 pounds. Such women may need a physician's help to maintain sufficient weight gain during pregnancy. For other women, the objective in weight control during pregnancy would be to keep weight gain reasonably close to the 20-to-25-pound average.

Drugs in Pregnancy

Recent years have brought an increased awareness of the importance of minimizing drug intake during pregnancy. Many drugs have been shown to increase the incidence of congenital defects; in fact, many physicians discourage the use of any nonessential drugs.

In general, the greatest risk of damage occurs during the first three months of pregnancy. Unfortunately, during much of this time, a woman may not know with any certainty that she is actually pregnant. Thus it is important to avoid drugs whenever pregnancy is suspected. This includes drugs of all types—street drugs, nonprescription drugstore remedies, and prescribed medications—unless the physician has specifically approved usage during pregnancy. It is important that any physician or dentist administering medications be told of the fact or possibility of pregnancy.

Smoking should also be avoided during pregnancy. The more a pregnant woman smokes, the less her baby will weigh at birth. As previously mentioned, the weight of a baby at birth is related to his chances of survival and helps determine how well he will thrive and develop during the first year of childhood.

Rh Factor in Pregnancy

The Rh factor is a chemical substance found in the red blood cells of about 85 percent of the American population. People who carry this substance are Rh positive (+); those who lack it are Rh negative (−). If, in any way, Rh+ blood enters the bloodstream of an Rh− person, the Rh factor stimulates the production of an antibody called *anti-Rh*. This antibody can destroy any red blood cells containing the Rh factor.

The Rh factor is of potential importance when an Rh− woman is pregnant with an Rh+ fetus (the father has to be Rh+). In such cases, the anti-Rh antibody may diffuse across the placenta from the mother's blood to the fetal blood where red blood cells may be destroyed. This is seldom a problem in the first such pregnancy (Rh− mother, Rh+ fetus), but may become quite serious by the second or third. The result is a severe form of anemia (*erythroblastosis fetalis*). The infant may be born dead or may die shortly after birth. If it survives, it may be mentally retarded.

In cases where tests during pregnancy indicate a dangerous anti-Rh level in the mother's blood, damage can often be prevented by transfusing the baby immediately after birth or even in the uterus before birth.

The sensitization of the Rh− mother (stimulation of her antibody production) does not usually take place during pregnancy, but at the time of delivery, miscarriage, or induced abortion of an Rh+ baby. Thus the problem can be prevented with a reverse vaccine (sold as RhoGAM and under other trade names). This vaccine (actually an injection of anti-Rh antibodies) will neutralize any Rh factor that might enter the mother's blood at the time of delivery of an Rh+ baby. The vaccine should be injected into an Rh− woman within 72 hours after such a delivery or after any miscarriage or induced abortion. This procedure protects the next pregnancy from Rh antibodies with over 90 percent effectiveness.

Sex in Pregnancy

A pregnant woman's sexual interest may increase, decrease, or remain virtually unchanged. Apparently the changes in hormone levels accompanying pregnancy have different effects on different women. In any case, sexual intercourse can usually be continued until delivery, unless some condition causes the physician to recommend against it. Intercourse should definitely be avoided in the event of abdominal or vaginal pain or discomfort, vaginal bleeding, or rupture of the membranes ("bag of waters"). Intercourse is usually avoided for a few weeks following delivery to allow the sexual organs to heal adequately.

Spontaneous Abortion (Miscarriage)

Many pregnancies terminate in a natural or spontaneous abortion (miscarriage). This is the expulsion of the embryo or fetus from the uterus before it has developed enough to survive on its own. About one of every ten diagnosed pregnancies terminates in this way. In addition, many spontaneous abortions occur so early in the pregnancy that the woman does not know with certainty of her pregnancy. Many early miscarriages are mistaken for late menstrual periods.

About 75 percent of spontaneous abortions occur within the first 12 weeks of the pregnancy. Common causes include death or abnormal development of the fetus, abnormalities of the uterus or placenta, and various diseases of the mother. Some women who experience repeated spontaneous abortions are found to have lower than normal levels of the hormone progesterone during early pregnancy. Such pregnancies can sometimes be saved by administering the deficient hormone.

Childbirth

Fetal Position

The first part of the fetal body seen in delivery is called the presenting part. When the head is lowermost—the usual case—it is a *cephalic presentation*; when the buttocks are lowermost, it is a *breech presentation* (Figure 6.7). Almost all babies are born with the back of the head appearing first.

Labor

Labor is the process by which the products of conception are expelled by the mother. The word *delivery* refers to the actual birth of the baby. This is expected to occur at *term*, or the end of the fortieth week.

Labor is divided into three stages: (1) preparatory stage, (2) birth of the baby, and (3) delivery of the afterbirth. The first stage starts with the beginning of labor contractions and lasts until the cervix of the uterus is fully dilated and ready for the passage of the child (Figure 6.8). The initial contractions are short, mild, and separated by intervals of ten to twenty minutes. The woman may walk around to remain comfortable between contractions. The discomfort usually starts in the small of the back and then sweeps around to the front of the abdomen. As labor progresses the contractions become more frequent (every three to five minutes), more intense, and longer lasting. The contractions preceding full dilation may be quite painful. The average duration of the first stage is about twelve hours for the first child and about eight hours for later children.

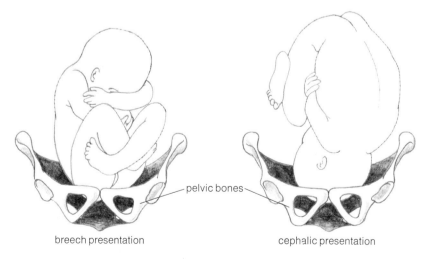

breech presentation   cephalic presentation

Figure 6.7 *The lowermost or presenting part of the fetus in delivery*

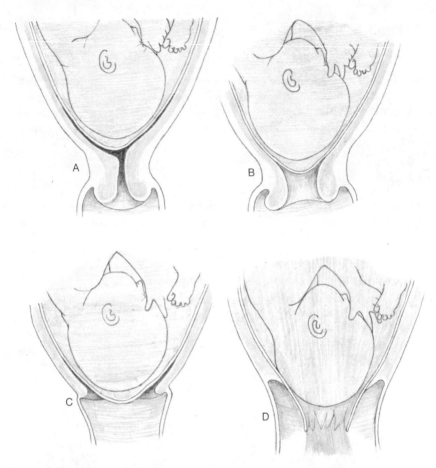

Figure 6.8 *Labor, first stage: (A) cervix before dilation, (B) beginning of dilation, (C) cervic fully dilated, and (D) rupture of the amnion*

Delivery starts with the full opening of the cervix and ends with the completed birth of the child (Figure 6.9). Contractions are severe and may last 50 to 100 seconds each, occurring at intervals of two or three minutes. The pressure of the contractions will usually cause the rupture of the amniotic sac ("bag of waters") during the early part of this stage (but sometimes before or during the first stage). During the contractions the mother strains and "bears down" strongly. When the cervix is open, the child begins to move down into the vagina. Each labor contraction moves the head down farther. With the cessation of each contraction, the head recedes somewhat. Just before the head emerges, it rotates to the side to pass the front part of the pelvic bone. With the next few contractions the neck and shoulders emerge. The body of the child is then quickly expelled. Immediately afterwards the remaining amniotic fluid gushes out. As soon as the child has emerged, the physician ties off the umbilical cord several

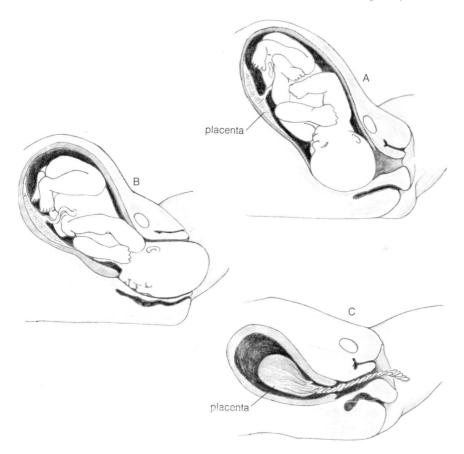

placenta

Figure 6.9 *Labor, first, second, and third stages: (A) end of first stage, cervix fully dilated, (B) second stage, presentation of head, and (C) third stage, separation from uterine wall and expulsion of placenta*

inches from the navel. Immediately after birth he assists the child to begin breathing. The child usually begins breathing within one minute and follows this with a strong cry. The average length of the second stage is 50 minutes in the first delivery and 20 minutes in later ones.

In the third stage contractions stop for a few moments following passage of the child and then begin again at regular intervals until the placenta is separated and expelled. Placental separation lasts about two to three minutes. Its expulsion from the uterus will take five to six additional minutes.

Reducing the Pain of Delivery

Normally the delivery of a child is painful. Discomfort can be reduced by preparing the mother. This preparation should include an understanding of the physical and emotional aspects of delivery. Learning controlled relaxation and breathing before delivery can reduce muscle spasms during labor. Such natural methods employed to reduce childbirth discomfort are referred to as *natural childbirth*.

Drugs are commonly used if the pain becomes too severe. Typical general anesthetics cause the woman to lose consciousness. Anesthetics injected into the spinal canal to deaden nerves coming from the uterus stop or diminish pain but leave the woman awake and aware. The particular drugs used depend on the woman's wishes and the physician's preference.

Complications of Delivery

Premature Birth

Occasionally a pregnancy ends before the fetus is mature. Whether the fetus survives will depend on what point during the pregnancy the termination occurs, the causes, and the conditions of the termination.

By definition, a premature infant is one born so early during the course of pregnancy that its organs have not reached full development. As a result, it has less chance to survive than a full-term infant. The most accurate guide to maturity is weight: a premature infant is one whose weight is 5½ pounds or less at delivery.

The less an infant weighs at birth, the less its chances of survival. The survival chance of a fetus at birth is often classified according to the following scale.

1 lb. 1 oz. or less	no chance of survival
1 lb. 2 oz. to 2 lb. 2 oz.	extremely poor chance of survival
2 lb. 3 oz. to 5 lb. 8 oz.	chances of survival range from poor to good according to weight
5 lb. 9 oz. or more	excellent chance of survival

In terms of age, the fetus may weigh 1 lb. 1 oz. during the sixth lunar month (22 weeks), or 2 lb. 3 oz. at end of the 28th week.

As many as half of all premature births cannot be explained. However, suspected maternal causes include high blood pressure, placental problems, and untreated syphilis. Prematurity is the leading cause of infant mortality (death between the time of birth and one year of age). The death of the infant may often be caused by respiratory difficulties or infections of various kinds.

Cesarean Section

The delivery of the fetus through an incision in the wall of the abdomen and uterus is a *cesarean section*.

About half of all cesarean sections are performed on women bearing their first child. The most frequent reason for cesarean section for a first delivery would be a space limitation—too large a child for the birth canal, a birth canal tumor, or abnormal pelvic structure. Other reasons might be a breech presentation, maternal diabetes, placental or umbilical cord complications. A cesarean section might also be performed in an attempt to save the fetus in the event a mother late in pregnancy is dying from other causes.

The other half of all cesarean sections are performed on women who have had a previous such delivery. In such cases the operation is performed to prevent rupture of the scar in the uterine wall, especially during labor. Although women who have experienced a previous cesarean section may give birth to a fetus through natural labor, subsequent deliveries are usually by cesarean section. Accordingly, how often a mother could deliver in this manner would depend upon the counsel of her physician. Most commonly a mother is advised to limit her children to two or three, although some women have had more cesarean sections.

Extrauterine Pregnancies

Some pregnancies develop outside the uterus, almost always in the fallopian tubes. This type of pregnancy is believed to be caused by slowed movement of the egg down the tube and by increased receptivity of the tube to the egg. Regardless of where the egg lodges, the embryo usually aborts. The mother may feel severe abdominal pains and, if hemorrhaging occurs, may show vaginal bleeding. In any event, the affected tube must be removed. This does not preclude later pregnancies, since one fallopian tube is still available for egg transport.

Induction of Labor

Where a pregnancy has developed medical complications, it may be necessary to terminate the pregnancy artificially in order to save the life of the fetus, the mother, or both. In a few cases a physician may decide to terminate the pregnancy for reasons of convenience—a mother who has had a history of rapid deliveries and who might not make it to the hospital in time, or who lives a great distance from a hospital. The timing and technique used to induce labor may present hazards to both the fetus and mother and must be decided only by a qualified physician.

Multiple Pregnancies

A *multiple pregnancy* is one in which the uterus contains two or more embryos. Twins occur in about 1 out of every 86 pregnancies, and triplets in about 1 out of every 7000 births.

Twins may result from the fertilization of either two separate eggs or a single egg. Twins developing from two separate eggs are called *fraternal* twins. Since they are from two separate eggs, fertilized by two separate sperm, they are the same as two different individuals developing at the same time. They may or may not share the same placenta (Figure 6.10).

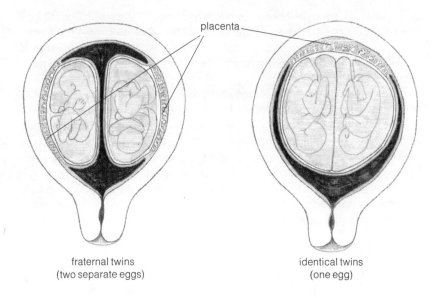

fraternal twins   identical twins
(two separate eggs)   (one egg)

Figure 6.10   *Development of twins*

Fraternal twins may be of the same or opposite sex and do not necessarily resemble each other more than other children of the same parents.

In about one out of every three cases of twins, one mature egg, fertilized by a single sperm, completely divides into two halves. Since both developing embryos are from the same egg and are fertilized by the same sperm, they are both *identical*, or alike genetically.

Triplets may arise from one, two, or three eggs. If from one egg, the egg has completely divided into three parts, in which case the triplets are identical. If from two eggs, one of the eggs has divided into two halves. Two of the triplets are identical and the other fraternal. The same would hold true for quadruplets, quintuplets, or other kinds of multiple pregnancies. In one case (the Dionne quintuplets) it is believed that all five were from a single egg and thus identical.

Current treatment of sterility due to lack of ovulation, using human gonadotropins, has not only successfully induced ovulation, but has also produced multiple eggs, often two or three. The common result has been multiple pregnancies. Efforts are being made to reduce this side effect.

Changes in the Mother after Delivery

By the end of the first week after delivery, the tissues of the vagina and uterus have greatly contracted. Within six weeks, the uterus is virtually back to normal. The abdominal wall ought to be back to original shape and firmness within two to three months.

Loss of Weight

With delivery a weight loss of around 11 pounds occurs. Within the next several weeks the mother should lose an additional 4½ to 5½ pounds. Unless she has gained excessively during pregnancy, she should return to her nonpregnant weight within six to eight weeks.

Menstruation

Women who do not nurse their babies usually menstruate within eight weeks after delivery. If the woman does nurse, menstruation is often delayed until the fifth or sixth month, although it may vary from 2 to 18 months. It may return before or after the breasts stop producing milk, and the first menstrual cycles may be irregular. Although ovulation is normally suspended while milk is produced, a nursing mother may become pregnant even though she has not yet menstruated since delivery.

Breasts

Breasts begin enlarging early in pregnancy, when they may produce small amounts of colostrum, a yellowish fluid. On about the third day after delivery, the breasts become engorged (filled) with milk. At first they may feel uncomfortable, but within several days these feelings disappear as production becomes regulated. Frequent and complete emptying of the breasts stimulates production. If the baby cannot empty the breasts in the early days of nursing, it is sometimes necessary to empty the breasts artificially. The length of time a mother breast-feeds her child will vary. Discontinuance of nursing should be a gradual process to allow milk production to decrease.

If a mother chooses not to nurse her baby, milk production can be suppressed by stopping the production of milk-producing hormones. Failure to remove accumulated milk from the breasts will also inhibit further milk production. However, the breasts will become engorged with milk in the meantime and this may cause some discomfort for several days.

Summary

I. Pregnancy—The Beginning

  A. Fertilization

    1. Egg viable for day or two after ovulation

    2. Fertilization usually in upper part of oviduct

    3. Fertilized egg called zygote

  B. Implantation

    1. Attachment of zygote to uterine lining

    2. Occurs several days after fertilization

   3. Placenta transfers nutrients from mother to child and wastes from child
   to mother

   4. No connection between bloodstreams of mother and child

  C. Amniotic fluid

   1. Contained in membranes surrounding embryo

   2. Protects embryo from injury, collects embryonic wastes

  D. Amniocentesis

   1. Sample of amniotic fluid withdrawn through needle

   2. Fluid and fetal cells may be examined for:

   a. Genetic defects

   b. Sex of child

  E. Determination of sex

   1. Determined by sex chromosomes: X and Y

   2. Normal female: 2 X chromosomes per cell (XX)

   3. Normal male: 1 X and 1 Y per cell (XY)

   4. Sperm determines sex of child:

   a. X-bearing sperm produces daughter

   b. Y-bearing sperm produces son

II. Typical Pregnancy

  A. Full-term pregnancy about 266 days from conception

  B. Diagnosis of pregnancy

   1. Common symptoms include:

   a. Missed menstrual period

   b. Increased size and sensitivity of breasts

   c. Nausea and vomiting

   d. Need for frequent urination

   2. Variety of pregnancy tests in use

   3. Positive diagnosis by fetal heartbeat, fetal movements, and appearance of
   fetal skeleton in X rays

  C. Prenatal care

   1. Care of pregnant woman and unborn baby

   2. Extremely important to mother and baby

  D. Morning sickness—nausea common in early pregnancy

E. Diseases in pregnancy

    1. German measles (rubella) during first six months may cause fetal defects

    2. Syphilis may infect fetus later in pregnancy

    3. Gonorrhea may infect eyes of baby at delivery

F. Toxemias

    1. Common in last three months of pregnancy

    2. Body retains salt and fluid

    3. Serious results if not adequately treated

G. Diet in pregnancy

    1. Must include plenty of proteins, vitamins, minerals

    2. Ideal weight gain usually 20 to 25 pounds

H. Drugs in pregnancy

    1. Drugs of all kinds to be avoided in early pregnancy

    2. Greatest risk of fetal damage during first three months

    3. Should avoid smoking in pregnancy

I. Rh factor in pregnancy

    1. Potential problem when Rh− mother carries Rh+ babies

    2. She produces antibodies that attack red blood cells of second or subsequent babies

    3. Causes severe anemia in baby (erythroblastosis fetalis)

    4. Problems prevented by injection of RhoGAM following birth of Rh+ baby to Rh− mother or after any spontaneous or induced abortion of Rh− woman

J. Sex in pregnancy

    1. Intercourse usually may be continued until delivery unless contraindicated

    2. Following delivery, intercourse is usually avoided for a few weeks to allow healing

K. Spontaneous abortion (miscarriage)

    1. Very common

    2. 75 percent in first 12 weeks of pregnancy

    3. Causes include fetal abnormalities, diseases of mother, low progesterone level

III. Childbirth

A. Fetal position—normally head first

B. Labor—three stages:

 1. First stage—from beginning of uterine contractions until cervix fully dilated

 2. Second stage—birth of the child

 3. Third stage—expulsion of placenta (afterbirth)

C. Reducing pain of delivery—natural methods and drugs

D. Complications of delivery

 1. Premature birth—5½ pounds or less

 2. Cesarean section

  a. Surgical delivery through abdominal wall

  b. Causes include fetal position, mother's pelvic structure, other maternal problems

 3. Extrauterine pregnancies

  a. Usually in fallopian tube

  b. Must be aborted

 4. Induction of labor—may terminate pregnancy early for variety of reasons

IV. Multiple Pregnancies

 A. May result from one or more eggs

 B. Twins from one egg called identical

 C. Twins from two eggs called fraternal

 D. May be result of fertility drugs

V. Changes in the Mother after Delivery

 A. Loss of weight

 B. Menstruation

  1. Within 8 weeks if not nursing

  2. In 2 to 18 months if nursing

  3. A nursing mother may become pregnant before menstruation

 C. Breasts

  1. Nursing stimulates milk production

  2. Breasts may be uncomfortable until production is regulated to consumption

  3. If not nursing baby, can suppress milk production with hormones and by accumulation of milk in breasts

Questions for Review

1. Where does fertilization usually occur?

2. What is amniocentesis and what is its value?

3. How is the sex of a baby determined?

4. What should be stressed in the diet of the pregnant woman?

5. Under what circumstances can the Rh factor complicate pregnancy? How can this problem be minimized?

6. What are the three stages of labor?

7. Distinguish between fraternal and identical twins.

8. Can a nursing mother become pregnant?

9. What is the importance of good prenatal care?

Chapter 7

NONMARITAL SEXUAL ADJUSTMENT

The sexual behavior of the unmarried person has always been a source of concern in our culture. For many years, the only acceptable form of sexual expression was intercourse between marriage partners. This absolute standard was, of course, unrealistic because the biological sex drive of an unmarried person is no different from that of a married person of the same age.

This restriction of sex to marriage has forced millions of people into marriage who really should have remained single. Additional millions have been forced to marry years before they were really ready, but at an age when their sexual drive was at a level they could not ignore.

Today, American society is hardly unanimous in what it considers right or wrong on matters of sexual conduct. During the past 50 or 60 years there has been a definite liberalization in the general attitude toward sex. But individual codes of behavior still range from total sexual freedom to strict prohibition of nonmarital sexual contact. Today, as always, unmarried individuals and couples must still decide on their own course of sexual conduct.

In this chapter, we will consider some of the psychological, sociological, and ethical aspects of various forms of sexual expression outside marriage. The decision of whether or not to engage in a particular form of sexual behavior is, for a mature person, a personal decision to be made after thoroughly considering all relevant information. Beyond that, it is the right and responsibility of the individual to make his or her own decisions.

Petting

There are various degrees of sexual relationship. One is *petting*, which might be defined as all relations more intimate than kissing but short of vaginal intercourse. Petting typically includes manual or oral stimulation, or both, of the breasts and sexual organs, and it may or may not lead to orgasm in either the male or female.

Oral stimulation involves much personal preference. To some people it is extremely enjoyable; to others it is equally unpleasant. It is most important that oral sex (or any other practice) not be forced upon a partner who does not really enjoy it.

Any value judgment regarding petting should be based on such considerations as the age and emotional maturity of each individual and their individual attitudes and backgrounds. Petting is a normal step in the development of psychosexual maturity and enables one to learn his own sexual responses and those of the opposite sex.

Petting does more to stimulate sexual desire than relieve sexual tensions. Petting is sexually arousing; the natural tendency in petting is to gradually become more and more intimate until it culminates in actual sexual intercourse. Consequently, the sexually aroused couple finds it very difficult to stop short of true intercourse. It is such unplanned intercourse that most often results in nonmarital pregnancy, since adequate contraception has not been considered or may not be readily available. Many couples develop techniques of petting to mutual orgasm as an alternative to intercourse. If this is to be done, it is important that no semen be allowed near the vaginal opening, since pregnancy can occur even without actual vaginal penetration by the penis.

Nonmarital Sexual Intercourse

Nonmarital sexual intercourse is a subject of considerable interest today. It is apparent that in the past few years there has been some increase in its prevalence and a great increase in its discussion. People now enter into nonmarital relationships more openly than at any time in the past. Despite improved contraceptive methods, the illegitimacy rate is at an all-time high, a good indication of increased nonmarital sexual activity.

As with petting, there are no universal answers to questions of whether or when to engage in nonmarital intercourse. Many individual factors must be considered. For some, religious beliefs dictate a definite NO if the tenets of their religion are to be followed. For others, below the age of consent, state laws dictate a firm NO. But, for the young adult, of legal age and holding no strong religious beliefs, it becomes a highly individual question, to be decided on the basis of personal values and philosophy, giving due consideration to all possible (positive and negative) results of such action. Some of the considerations that should be included in making a decision about nonmarital sex follow.

Pregnancy

The basic motivation behind most of the legal, religious, and social regulations pertaining to marriage is to provide a stable family environment for the child and to determine who is responsible for its support. Even today, although attitudes toward sex have changed considerably, pregnancy out of marriage is regarded as a serious problem by many people.

Modern contraceptive methods can greatly reduce the chance of pregnancy. Anyone engaging in nonmarital sexual relations should choose a highly effective contraceptive method and be certain that it is used properly. Even though a normally foolproof method (such as pills) is chosen, the couple should plan and agree on the action to be taken in case accidental pregnancy occurs. If a couple is not mature enough to discuss this problem realistically, then it is questionable whether they are mature enough to engage in sexual relations at all. Some of the paths available are given below.

ABORTION

Some precautions are in order if abortion is the chosen solution. An induced abortion temporarily interferes with the body's hormonal system, and some women may need postabortion medical help. Repeated induced abortions may later lead to the inability to conceive or carry a child to full term. For some, religious or personal philosophical viewpoints may raise emotional or ethical questions that need to be answered. Although nearly all abortions are warranted, abortion should not be viewed as a substitute for the individual's use of a reliable contraceptive.

SINGLE PARENTHOOD

The prospect of keeping and raising a child out of wedlock holds little appeal for many women. Yet in recent years increasing numbers of unmarried women are taking this option. Actually, single parenthood probably better serves the welfare of both the mother and the child than marrying "to give the kid a name" and then enduring the bitterness of eventual divorce.

MARRIAGE

Although pregnancy is one of the commonest reasons for getting married, it may be one of the poorest. A high percentage of forced marriages turn into disasters, leading to divorce or, perhaps even worse, to meaningless, bitter coexistence. Unless both parties truly want to marry, it is far better to take one of the other options.

ADOPTION

In many cases adoption is the best course of action, because it should assure the child of a loving home where it is welcomed rather than resented. There is currently a strong demand for newborn infants for adoption.

Venereal Disease

The risk of venereal disease depends on the pattern of nonmarital sexual relationships. If the only relationship involved is between a mutually faithful couple then, of course, there is no risk of venereal disease (assuming neither is infected to start with). If a person has many casual sexual contacts or has intercourse with anyone who does have such contacts, then the risk of venereal disease is greatly increased; syphilis and gonorrhea are now epidemic.

Psychological Motivation

A multitude of subtle factors motivate the expression of sexuality, in addition to the more obvious need for release from sexual tensions. These nonsexual motives are not always undesirable, since they are generally present to some extent in any sexual relationship, within or outside of marriage. Among the more universal motives in sexuality are the need to feel wanted as a sexual partner (sexually attractive) and successful as a lover. The ego reinforcement obtained through successful sexual relationships is very important for the total emotional adjustment of most adults. The expression of love is another useful nonsexual function of sexuality. Among the less desirable sexual motives is the use of sex for bargaining power, where sexual privileges are traded for various emotional and/or material rewards and withheld as punishment for failure of the partner to provide such rewards. Another misuse of sex is as a trap to force an expression of commitment from a partner who does not really feel any great degree of love.

It is important for each sexual partner to understand the motives of the other. If it is going to be "pure" sex (sex for physical satisfaction alone), then both partners should share this feeling, and no pretense of love or other commitment should be made. Deception amounts to exploitation and can only lead to someone feeling used and hurt.

Effect on Future Marriage

One of the traditional concerns about nonmarital sex has been whether it might affect the success of any future marriage. This is really a very difficult question to answer, for several reasons. First, so many factors relate to marital happiness that it is really impossible to determine cause and effect. In addition, it is fruitless to make statistical comparisons of the divorce rate, orgasm rate, or any other "indicator" of marital happiness between groups who have had and have not had premarital sexual experience. The problem is that people who have nonmarital sex also differ statistically in many other ways from those who do not. For example, they tend to have more permissive attitudes on all phases of sexuality, are more likely to use alcohol, tobacco, and marijuana, are less likely to hold strong religious beliefs, and feel less bound by the traditional sanctity of marriage. If one wants to "prove" that premarital sex has either a positive or a negative effect on future marital success, it is easy to find statistical studies to support either point of view. In reality, few of these studies can be considered valid, since it is impossible to separate nonmarital sex habits from all the other associated habits and attitudes. About the only safe conclusion is that premarital sexual experience seems neither essential nor detrimental to marital happiness.

Social Considerations

As noted earlier, different societies and different elements within one society hold varying attitudes toward nonmarital sexual intercourse, ranging from total permissiveness to total prohibition. In the United States, we find an ambiguous situation, with many people disapproving the sexual activities of others but excusing their own similar activities. The "official" attitude here is prohibitive toward sexual activity before marriage. The "unofficial" attitude is still the highly discredited double standard, which is much more tolerant toward the sexual activities of men than of women. This is an unfortunate carry-over from the era when women were not expected to enjoy sexual intercourse and were expected to be subservient to men.

Fear of discovery drives many couples to seek less than ideal places for their sexual relationships, often with unhappy results. The fear, anxiety, and haste may make orgasm impossible for the female, thus building a negative attitude toward sex. After several disappointing, frustrating experiences she may feel that she is sexually inadequate or that she is being exploited for the purely selfish satisfaction of the male.

Legal Considerations

In a few states any sexual intercourse between unmarried persons is illegal, but such laws are seldom, if ever, enforced. Of more importance are laws that prohibit intercourse with a woman below the age of consent, which varies among the states from 14 to 21, but is most often 18 years of age. A male having intercourse with a girl below this age can be prosecuted for statutory rape, a felony offense. Even if a girl appears to be older and lies about her age, the male can still be convicted.

Still another problem can arise when an unmarried girl becomes pregnant and sues for child support. Any male who has had intercourse with her during a given period of time may be named in the suit.

Prostitution

Prostitution is the exchange of sexual favors for a fee—usually promiscuously and without affection. While the most common form of prostitution is female and heterosexual, there also exists male heterosexual prostitution as well as male and female homosexual prostitution. The distinction between prostitution and amateur sex is sometimes vague, as when a woman exchanges sexual favors for her personal gain, such as job advancement, or accepts expensive gifts or living expenses from a wealthy male friend.

Prostitution is illegal throughout most of the United States. It is often singled out as a prime example of victimless crime since it involves a mutually agreed-upon exchange of fee for service rendered between two consenting persons. Both enter into the relationship voluntarily and, theoretically, both benefit. Those who favor the prohibition of prostitution usually cite as their grounds religious beliefs, fear of organized crime, suppression of venereal diseases, degradation of women to a commodity, and the possibility of robbery and blackmail under the guise of prostitution.

Masturbation

Masturbation is the production of orgasm by self-stimulation of the sex organs. Despite the elaborate mythology about the supposedly harmful effects of masturbation, it is now recognized as a harmless and normal part of sexuality in both the male and the female. Over 90 percent of all males masturbate at some time in their lives, as do over 60 percent of all females. Masturbation is quite common among married as well as single people.

The old wives' tale that masturbation leads to insanity probably originated in the fact that emotionally disturbed individuals sometimes masturbate excessively in a retreat from reality.

Masturbation may begin at any age. The frequency of masturbation varies considerably, from once a month to several times daily. Females typically masturbate less frequently than males. Therapists sometimes recommend masturbation to women as a way of learning their sexual responses, building positive feelings about sex, and becoming more orgasmic.

Alternate Lifestyles

Increasing numbers of people are choosing to live in some arrangement other than traditional marriage. They are generally motivated by a search for individual freedom and fulfillment. Actually, most of these lifestyles are not really new at all, but have long existed in various forms and at various periods of history. In many cases, though, the motivations behind these alternate lifestyles are new, and in almost every case the openness of these arrangements and their acceptance by society is growing.

Certainly the simplest alternate lifestyle is just to remain single and live alone. If a person is satisfied with this arrangement, then there is no psychological or sociological reason why he or she should not pursue it.

Long-term homosexual "marriage" is another possibility, and for many individuals proves to be satisfactory. As is true for several other lifestyles, persons choosing homosexual marriage should be strong enough to withstand the stigma, however unwarranted it may be, that some elements of our society still direct toward certain lifestyles.

The alternate lifestyle that has attracted the greatest following in recent years is the common practice of "living together," which in many respects resembles the old-fashioned common-law marriage. In this arrangement, a heterosexual couple sets up housekeeping in a fashion that greatly resembles marriage, the principal difference being the absence of license or ceremony. The motivations for living together are what distinguishes this as a separate lifestyle. While old-fashioned common-law marriage is often associated with lower income levels and is usually motivated by economic expediencies, living together is a middle- and upper-class phenomenon with various motivations. It may be based on a philosophic rejection of marriage as too confining and restrictive for individual growth. It may be motivated by the romantic view that the love relationship remains stronger when it is maintained voluntarily, rather than enforced by the legal contract of marriage. In still other cases, living together is viewed as a trial period which, if successful for a period of time, will lead to legal marriage.

Most couples living together expect of each other the same fidelity typical of marriage partners, with neither person free to engage in outside sexual relations or even to date. Thus the degree of freedom in the relationship of living together is really little greater than in marriage, with the exception of the legal ease with which the relationship can be terminated. Of course, the emotional trauma in breaking up can be as great as in terminating a marriage.

Even among the strongest advocates of living together, many feel that legal marriage should precede the birth of children. The commitment involved in legal marriage, while not guaranteeing a lasting relationship, at least indicates an intention on the part of each person to make a stable partnership. In addition, the great majority of people in our society still stigmatize the child born of unmarried parents. While this stigma is terribly unfair to the child, it is a reality that will probably last for some time.

The most revolutionary of the alternate life styles is group marriage—a catch-all term applied to a wide variety of polygamous living arrangements in which small groups of adult males and females, and their children, live together under one roof or in a close-knit settlement, calling themselves a family, tribe, commune, or community. Generally all property is collectively owned, and all the members work for the common good. Many group marriages represent utopian minisocieties largely opposed to the mores and values of contemporary American society.

The collectivism of group marriages usually extends to their sexual relationships. While some communes consist of conventionally faithful married couples, more commonly there is some degree of sexual sharing.

Most group marriages, as well as most other utopian schemes, are destined to fail. Many of the problems of traditional marriage are merely multiplied in group marriage. Considering the difficulty in finding a mere two people who can live together compatibly, it becomes a near impossibility to find larger groups of people who can live harmoniously and lovingly together. A marriage of one man and one woman involves one interrelationship, which is difficult to keep in working order. But the smallest possible group marriage, three people, involves 3 interrelationships; four people makes 6 relationships; and fifteen people results in 105 relationships. Jealousies and love conflicts are similarly multiplied in group marriages, and considerable individual freedom must be sacrificed in the process of coordinating and scheduling many lives. Thus most group marriages are unstable and typically last for only a few months.

Summary

I. Petting

   A. Relations more intimate than kissing, but short of vaginal coitus

   B. A normal step in development of psychosexual maturity

   C. Many couples pet to mutual orgasm

   D. Value judgments on petting should be based on age, emotional maturity, attitudes, and backgrounds of each individual

II. Nonmarital Sexual Intercourse

   A. Decision to engage in nonmarital intercourse an individual matter, based on personal values and philosophy

   B. Other considerations include:

      1. Pregnancy, with alternatives including

         a. Abortion

         b. Single parenthood—becoming increasingly common

         c. Marriage—usually a poor choice

         d. Adoption—strong demand for babies

      2. Venereal disease—risk depends on behavior

      3. Psychological motivations—intercourse often motivated by nonsexual needs

      4. Effect on future marriage—no definite answer

      5. Social considerations—attitudes vary

      6. Legal considerations

       a. Age of consent

       b. Possibility of child-support payments

III. Prostitution

  A. Sex for a fee

  B. Male or female, homosexual or heterosexual

  C. Illegal in most of United States

IV. Masturbation

  A. Production of orgasm by self-stimulation of sex organs

  B. A perfectly harmless part of normal male or female sexuality

V. Alternate Lifestyles

  A. Remaining single and living alone

  B. Long-term homosexual "marriage "

  C. Living together

  D. Group marriage

Questions for Review

1. What are some positive and negative values of petting?

2. In your opinion, who should engage in nonmarital intercourse?

3. What factors should a woman consider in contemplating single parenthood?

4. Why do marriages forced by unplanned pregnancy stand so little chance of success?

5. When is venereal disease a consideration in nonmarital intercourse?

6. What are some of the nonsexual motivations for sexual intercourse?

7. What is the "age of consent"?

8. Why have group marriages not been notably successful?

Chapter 8
MARRIAGE

People are still getting married. In fact, they are doing so in near-record numbers, despite the predictions the past few years that conventional marriage was on its last legs. While many rightfully choose not to marry, the majority of young people still have faith in the institution of marriage and are willing to try it, though perhaps in a form different from their parents' marriages.

At the same time that more people are marrying, a record number of existing marriages are ending in divorce. Many divorces represent marriages that should never have taken place—the seeds of failure were present at the time of the marriage. Marriage should be entered into rationally rather than emotionally. Both individuals should objectively evaluate their own readiness for marriage and the nature of their relationship.

Individual Readiness for Marriage

In many ways, readiness for marriage is a subjective quality. There is no single criterion of age or physical development or emotional make-up that qualifies one for matrimony. However, certain objective standards taken together may serve as an index of marital readiness.

Age at Marriage

More than any other characteristic, the age of the couple allows one to predict the success of the marriage: success increases with the age of the couple. Emotional conflict, sexual problems, money problems, in-law trouble, and divorce are all much more common among those couples who marry in their teens than among those who marry later. Marriages where the husband was in his teens are particularly unhappy.

The national average age at first marriage is about 23 years for men and 21 years for women. Reversing a trend of many years, the average age of marriage is increasing slightly. This statistic may reflect the increasing number of couples who live together before marrying.

One of the sources of problems with young marriages is that many people greatly change their value systems between the ages of 16 and 22. During this period, one's interests, tastes, ideals, standards, and goals usually change completely. If people marry before this change, there is a strong possibility that they will no longer meet each other's tastes and emotional needs.

A related problem is that early marriage often interferes with the development of a mature philosophy. There is a tendency for the intellectual growth of an individual to stop with marriage. This can be prevented, of course, but many young married people fall into a deep philosophical and intellectual rut from which they never escape. Often one partner grows while the other stagnates, a sure formula for unhappiness.

Emotional Maturity

The emotional demands of marriage are much greater than those a couple experiences during dating. Thus an important requirement for marriage is emotional maturity. Such maturity generally increases with age, but some individuals remain emotionally adolescent even though they have legally become adults.

Before marriage, a person should be as free as possible of emotional maladjustments such as moodiness, jealousy, anxiety, depression, and insecurity. These emotional states can destroy a marriage. A person subject to such maladjustment should seek qualified professional counsel.

The truly mature person has skill in establishing and maintaining good interpersonal relationships. He recognizes the needs of others and is willing to assume some responsibility for meeting these needs. Each partner in a marriage must have such a concern for the other if happiness is to result.

Social Maturity and Experience

Social maturity develops through social interaction. Before marriage, social maturity should be built through dating many different individuals. This gives a better basis for the selection of a marriage mate and helps satisfy social curiosity. The person whose dating is more restricted may later, after marriage, feel that he has missed something and try to compensate through extramarital affairs.

It is important to experience a period of single, independent life before marriage, a time of freedom between the dependence of living with one's parents and the responsibilities of marriage. It is only through living away from parents that one can really come to know oneself, develop full social competency, and learn to manage one's own affairs. A strong argument can be made that anyone who is too immature, insecure, or otherwise incompetent to live independently is, for the same reason, not ready for marriage. Many people, after enjoying their independence, feel a desire to "settle down" into marriage. Others find the single life permanently satisfying and prefer not to marry. There is absolutely no reason why anyone in the latter group should feel any obligation to marry.

Financial Resources

Although less important than the preceding personal characteristics, financial factors must be considered before marriage. The minimum amount of money a couple needs to live on varies greatly. Most young couples enter marriage without great amounts of money.

Often the parents of student couples offer some financial help, but the couple should evaluate this possibility in respect to their sense of independence. If such help is going to be a source of conflict, then some other financial arrangement must be developed. If the couple is to rely on the earnings of the wife, then obviously it is important that a highly reliable method of contraception be used. A pregnancy in this situation could be a serious financial and emotional burden.

Selecting for Happiness

Chances of a happy marriage are determined by one's own personal traits, those of one's chosen partner, and how those traits act upon each other. Consider, then, some of the traits to look for in a potential mate. Right away, let us dispel the notion of the "one and only" or the "marriage made in heaven." For every person there are thousands of potentially good mates. If the person you might be considering for marriage seems to have a serious deficiency in some respect, just keep looking. On the other hand, if no one seems to fit your ideal for marriage, you might well be overcritical or just not ready for marriage.

Positive Personality Traits

By far the most important characteristic in a potential marriage partner is his or her personality. Some people have positive personality traits that enable them to enjoy life to its fullest and to bring joy to anyone in contact with them. Others are so burdened with negative reactions that their own happiness is impossible, as is that of anyone who must live with them. Traits that help produce happiness in marriage include the ability to adjust easily to changes in conditions, optimism, a sense of humor, an honest concern for the needs of others, a sense of ethics, and the freedom from such negative traits as anxiety, depression, insecurity, and jealousy.

Mutual Need Satisfaction

The happy and lasting marriage is one in which the needs of each individual are adequately satisfied. While the idea may not appeal to romantics, the basic reason why people marry is to satisfy their needs. A good marriage satisfies many needs—sex, love, companionship, security, and subtle psychological needs. Since everyone is unique in his psychological needs, the characterization of the imaginary ideal partner for each person is a highly individual matter. Only through knowing each other very well, over a long period of time and in a variety of situations (both pleasant and unpleasant), can two people learn whether they are able to fulfill each other's needs.

Genuine Mutual Love

The distinction between genuine love and infatuation is not always clear. Infatuation is frequently associated with immaturity, a puppy love. It is a kind of substitute for love until a person has the capacity to love someone fully and deeply. It tends to involve sexual attraction more than personality attraction. Infatuation is unrealistic, a fantasy. The object of the infatuation is seen as a dream mate, lacking any undesirable traits. Infatuation is often immediate, whereas love develops with time. Infatuation often wears off quickly, yet it may, with time, develop into mature love.

A person truly in love is concerned with his or her loved one's happiness and well-being. He or she is tender, considerate, and constant; is willing to sacrifice some pleasures in order to bring pleasure to the loved one. There is a desire to share ideas, emotions, goals, and experiences. Love continues to grow indefinitely with the passage of time.

There should definitely be a strong sexual attraction between any persons considering marriage. It would be an unusual person who would want to marry in the absence of sexual attraction. However, many people mistake sexual attraction for love, when it is actually just part of love. A couple can have a very good sexual relationship without loving each other, but such a relationship would make a weak basis for a happy marriage.

Agreement on Parenthood

Any couple considering marriage should reveal their true feelings about having children. Ideally, they should agree on whether they want children and, if so, how many. It is always unfortunate when a person who wants children chooses a partner who would rather remain childless. Automatically, one or the other is destined to be unhappy. If there is serious disagreement on this matter, each individual should look for another mate.

Incidentally, if neither person wants children, there is no reason to feel guilty about a decision to remain childless. Studies have shown that children are not essential to happiness in marriages. In fact, they have been found to place additional strain on an already unhappy marriage. A couple need feel no obligation to themselves or to society to produce children.

Hereditary Traits

Some individuals carry obvious hereditary defects. Others seem perfectly normal, but come from families in which such defects are known to occur. The latter individuals may or may not be carrying undesirable hidden genes. If there is any question regarding the possibility of transmitting defective genes, it is wise to seek genetic counseling, either from a physician or a specially trained genetic counselor whom a physician may recommend. Any decision to marry and have children, marry and not have children, or not to marry at all should be based upon such advice and not on the advice of uninformed friends and relatives.

Similarity in Background

It is important for any couple considering marriage to take critical, objective look at their differences in general background. These differences may be minor and insignificant or major and have a great bearing on the marriage. Many studies have shown that the more similarities between two individuals, the greater their chances of marital success. Significant differences may involve age, nationality or ethnic background, economic status, education, intelligence, religion, or previous marital status. Most marriages can be successful, despite these differences, if the couple is willing to work out the special problems involved.

AGE

When there is a wide difference in age, one must examine why one wants to marry a person considerably older or younger. Is it the desire for immediate economic security? Is it the inability to find a partner close to one's age? Is it a feeling of flattery at commanding the attention of a more mature or more youthful person? Is the older person seen as a father or mother image? Does the older person need to dominate or the younger to be dominated? On the average, marriages are happiest when the man and wife are within a few years of each other in age. However, if the marriage with a wide age difference fulfills the needs of each person, then such a marriage may be quite happy.

ETHNIC DIFFERENCES

Marriages between members of different ethnic groups may face the most difficult problems of any type of mixed marriage. Not only can there be problems within the marriage, but the couple may experience resentment and prejudice from both family members and outsiders.

The internal problems in these marriages may revolve around customs, standards, and points of view. For example, the attitudes toward women and their rights, duties, and status may be quite different. Family patterns of authority and the role expected of each member may conflict. Attitudes on raising children and care of elderly relatives may be another area of disagreement. These problems do not appear in all mixed marriages, but such topics should be discussed objectively before marriage.

The problems caused by the prejudices of family members and society are particularly frustrating, because they should not exist in an enlightened society. The source of many of these problems is the ethnocentric attitude of groups that guard their ethnic heritage to excess and often sincerely believe in the supremacy of their group over all others. The elders of some of these groups encourage their youth to maintain a distance from outsiders, to continue to respect the traditions and customs of the group, and to marry within the group. The young man or woman who marries outside the group may be rejected even by the immediate family.

Other problems may arise in finding housing and employment, especially in black-white marriages. There may even be problems in finding friends who will fully accept both partners. The amount of social prejudice felt by the couple will vary from city to city and with the part of the country. Ethnically mixed couples may find their best acceptance today in college towns, where the general attitude is usually more enlightened and liberal than in many other places.

It is likely that the number of mixed marriages will continue to increase, if the trends of the past few years can be projected into the future. The breakdown of social prejudices is painfully slow, but it can be hoped that the need for a discussion such as this will eventually be a thing of the past.

ECONOMIC STATUS

Even though our society has always claimed that one of its goals is social equality regardless of economic status, patterns of behavior do vary greatly with economic level. Behavior that is "correct" at one economic level may meet with disapproval at another level. Attitudes toward authority, freedom, ethics, education, and other values may differ. Marriage of individuals of different economic backgrounds may require some adjustment of these attitudes.

EDUCATION

Even with the increasing educational opportunities available today, it is not unusual for a young couple to have a wide difference in level of education. Changes in values, personal goals, and social sophistication usually accompany a greater extent of education. Compatibility in marriage is largely a matter of common interests, and differently educated persons are likely to have few common interests. There is a tendency for boredom to develop, and for both to go their own ways.

Yet there are individuals who, though short on formal education, have horizons wider than many college graduates who have confined their interests to a specialized major field of study.

INTELLIGENCE

Perhaps a similarity in level of intelligence is even more important than similarity in level of education. In marriages with a wide contrast in basic intelligence, the partners tend to drift apart. Not only may the more intelligent partner long for stimulating exchange of ideas with someone else, but also the less intelligent person may develop feelings of inferiority. Each may grow lonely. These marriages can be successful if each partner recognizes the other's strong points and allows each to excel individually.

RELIGION

Religious differences can be one of the most disruptive influences in a marriage. The important factor is not simply the difference in religious affiliation, but the significance the individuals attach to their beliefs. To some, religion means nothing. To others, it is the unifying force in their lives. A religion shared in marriage can form a powerful bond between husband and wife. Religious conflict can act as a powerful wedge, forcing them far apart.

Most of the differences we have thus far discussed can be worked out satisfactorily. However, in certain combinations of religious beliefs, if each person remains faithful to his religion, there may be constant conflict throughout the marriage. Such marriages should be entered into only after the couple have reached mutually acceptable answers to all possible questions and problems of mixed-marriage life. Nothing should be left to chance or to be settled after marriage. The couple should go together to discuss their decisions with the parents and the clergy of each faith. Their decisions should be clearly in mind and well stated (in writing, if possible), so there can be no possibility of a misunderstanding. If, after such dis-cusscions with parents and clergy, there still seem to be conflicts, it would probably be better for each to look for someone whose religious beliefs are more similar to his own. This may seem to be a pessimistic view of the problem, but it does seem that the best way to avoid the problems of a religiously incompatible marriage is to avoid the marriage itself.

Danger Signals in a Relationship

Many people are married only a short time before they realize that their marriages are mistakes. As a result, the divorce rate is very high during the first few years of marriage. It is obvious that many divorces are the result of the wrong people getting married in the first place. Much misery could be prevented if such incompatible couples could be identified before they made the commitment of marriage. The following characteristics of the premarital relationship signal danger.

QUARRELING

Quarreling is a very serious danger signal in any relationship moving toward marriage. Such quarreling is almost certain to continue after marriage, probably at an escalated frequency and intensity. Quarreling almost always means that the needs of one or both partners are not being fulfilled in their relationship. As long as needs are mutually met, there is no need to quarrel, and a relationship runs smoothly. Couples must not rely on the folk belief, so often reinforced by movies, television, novels, and other media, that true love seldom runs smoothly and that they should not be concerned over their "lovers' quarrels." The theme of lovers fighting, breaking up, making up, marrying, and living happily ever after occurs frequently in the entertainment media, but very rarely in real life. Constant quarreling calls for serious evaluation, in which the real reasons for the quarrels are determined through open and honest communication of feelings. If an area of conflict cannot be clearly resolved, it would seem foolish for a couple to marry.

LACK OF COMMUNICATION

If either partner cannot openly and freely express his feelings on any subject to the other, this casts considerable doubt on their chances of a happy marriage. Not only is lack of communication a problem in itself, but it can also be an outward symptom of a personality problem in one of the individuals or a basic incompatibility of the two. It is important that any couple considering marriage thoroughly discuss their feelings about sex (roles, frequency, techniques, etc.), parenthood, contraception, family finances, role of each partner in a marriage, in-law relationships, and general lifestyle. Any inability to communicate or open disagreement in one of these areas can only be interpreted as a danger sign and portent of an unhappy marriage.

LACK OF CONFIDENCE THAT THE MARRIAGE WILL BE GOOD

Another prime indicator of unhappy marriage is doubts by either partner that the marriage is likely to succeed. Retrospective surveys of married couples have shown that the happiest married couples are those who had the fewest doubts before marriage that they would be happy. In contrast, a large percentage of unhappily married couples recall serious premarital doubts abut the ultimate success of their marriages.

OFF-AGAIN, ON-AGAIN RELATIONSHIPS

A history of temporary breakups in a relationship is strongly predictive of failure in marriage. Such breakups indicate that one or both partners may lack a strong commitment to the relationship, that needs are not being well fulfilled, or that other serious problems exist. The same problems that cause temporary breakups are likely to remain after marriage, leading to continued trouble. Couples with a history of breakups should carefully consider the underlying causes before entering into marriage.

Premarital Counseling

Increased emphasis is being placed on premarital counseling to assist couples in making an adequate marital adjustment. It has been found that the probability of happiness in marriage can be predicted by examining certain background factors, personality traits, engagement relations, engagement adjustment, and other anticipated factors.

The counselor may be a professional marriage counselor, a clergyman, or a physician. Some marriage counselors use personality tests to indicate a person's suitability for marriage or the couple's likely compatibility. The couple should discuss with the counselor any fears or inhibitions they may have regarding sex. He should question them regarding financial plans, housing, budgets, and any other phase of marriage that may be subject to adjustment.

Even though a state law may require only a blood test for syphilis, each prospective partner should have a thorough physical examination to detect any condition that might interfere with sexual relations, childbearing, or earning a living. There should be a consultation with a gynecologist regarding the preferred method of contraception for the couple.

Marital Sexual Adjustment

A sexually inexperienced bride and groom may very likely have some anxieties about their wedding night. Each partner hopes for a mutually satisfactory sexual experience, but may have many doubts. Much of this anxiety can be reduced with proper preparation. The bride's premarital consultation with a gynecologist can help considerably. At that time a contraceptive method should be prescribed which minimizes the fear of pregnancy and which will not interfere with total abandon in sexual expression. Oral contraceptives and IUD's are ideal for this purpose. The gynecologist should also check a virginal bride-to-be for the presence of an unusually tough hymen. Such a hymen can make her sexual initiation painful and unpleasant. It is a simple matter for the gynecologist to dilate or cut such a hymen, thus eliminating the possibility of a painful introduction to marital sex.

Even with these precautions, a couple should not expect their first sexual experiences to be entirely satisfactory. An inexperienced groom may seldom have adequate sexual control and, on the first attempt at intercourse, may ejaculate and lose erection almost immediately after vaginal penetration, or even before. But after a few minutes, he should be able to attain erection again and, with seminal pressure reduced, delay ejaculation for some time.

An inexperienced bride may be disappointed in her failure to achieve orgasm on her wedding night. But many studies have shown that a virgin bride often does not reach orgasm through intercourse for a matter of several days, weeks, or even months. In fact, a significant number of women achieve orgasm only after a year or more. Marital adjustments take time. Time is required to break down fears and inhibitions and to learn sexual techniques. Open communication of sexual feelings by both persons is especially important.

Sexual satisfaction is not the only aim of marriage. The success of a marriage cannot be measured by the number of orgasms per month, as some of the handbooks to marital sex seem to indicate. Sex must be viewed as only a part of marriage. On the other hand, a couple should not neglect working toward a satisfying sexual adjustment.

Extramarital Sexual Relations

A majority of Americans still consider sexual exclusiveness in marriage an important value. At the time of marriage, most people plan to remain faithful and expect their new mates to do the same. Yet recent surveys show that infidelity occurs at some time in over half of all marriages. Thus there seems to be a definite gap between what we believe (or say we believe) and what we actually practice.

Often it is difficult to pinpoint the real causes of infidelity, because most people try to justify their behavior with elaborate rationalizations. Though infidelity is often attributed to an unsatisfactory sexual relationship within a marriage, it also occurs when the marital sexual adjustment is entirely satisfactory. In fact, the real motivations for infidelity are probably more often nonsexual than sexual. Among the more common reasons given for infidelity are boredom with the marital partner or the home situation in general, lack of sexual interest by or in the marital partner, and lack of warmth, love, or affection in or for the partner. Some people even rationalize their extramarital affairs as evidence of their true love for their partner, since their affairs enable them to remain married and to tolerate both the marriage and the spouse. Some people explain their infidelity on the simple basis of a healthy heterosexual interest in a variety of partners. This is, of course, part of the philosophy of the so-called swinger.

The amount of guilt associated with infidelity varies greatly. Those most bothered by guilt would be people whose behavior contradicts their own values and standards. But guilt presents little or no problem for many people, sometimes because there are no conflicting values to produce it. Others so thoroughly rationalize their infidelity that they escape all guilt. For many people, the worst psychological problem associated with infidelity is some degree of anxiety related to a fear of getting caught by either their own or their paramour's spouse, an unpleasant situation at best.

When the rationalizations are stripped away, three principal causes of infidelity emerge. All are interrelated, and all reveal an underlying inability to be fully committed to a relationship of love and mutual regard and respect. It is a mistake to always assign the blame to the partner who is unfaithful, as the problem may involve characteristics in the supposedly innocent partner that almost force the infidelity of the other as a matter of ego preservation. Thus the problem may lie in either partner or in both. Any lasting relationship requires commitments and compromises that one or both partners may be unable or unwilling to make. The three basic problems (after Leon Salzman, in *Medical Aspects of Human Sexuality*, February 1972) include:

1. *Lack of commitment.* Some people marry even though their degree of love and commitment is uncertain. Such marriages may be motivated by financial, social, religious, or psychological factors. An often-expressed attitude is, "Well, if it doesn't work out, I can always get a divorce." Any expectation of fidelity in such a case is totally unjustified. Obviously, anyone so weakly committed should avoid marriage.

2. *Failure in adjustment.* Marriages in this category begin in love, loyalty, and commitment, but the partners gradually drift apart, until one or both must go outside the marriage in order to fulfill emotional needs. A cause of such problems may be the unrealistic expectations that so many people hold for marriage. Almost from birth, we are conditioned by various media and the national folklore to expect to marry and live happily ever after. The ideal marriage is portrayed as a state of perpetual euphoria in which problems just don't exist. Sex is supposed to be supremely enjoyable, with both partners always in the mood for sex at the same times and each sexual act ending in earthshaking orgasms, each bigger and better than ever before. Nonsense. In every marriage there are going to be problems: money problems, in-law problems, sexual problems, illnesses, child-raising problems, role and identity problems, conflicting interests, conflicting careers, and, if the marriage lasts that long, problems of aging and retirement. When the realities of married life are compared with the unrealistic expectations that most of us hold, then even a very good marriage can look like a dismal failure. In our disappointment, we feel entirely justified in going outside of marriage to satisfy our various needs. Into this category fall the millions of people who excuse their infidelity on the basis that it sustains their marriage.

3. *Personality disorders.* A variety of personality structures make fidelity impossible. Included are the sociopathic, the paranoid, the jealous, the immature, and the egocentric types. A very common trait associated with infidelity is insecurity about one's sexual attractiveness or adequacy. The person who has numerous short-term affairs is often motivated by a need for reassurance that he or she can attract lovers and perform well sexually.

In conclusion, it seems that while infidelity is occasionally part of a neurotic or psychotic personality development, it more often represents a rational and understandable form of behavior in a normal person. It may occur in people who are basically loyal and faithful, in response to compelling emotional needs. It may occur as a single brief affair, as a series of occasional brief affairs, or as a chronic situation.

While the incidence of infidelity has traditionally been higher in men than among women, this is believed to have been the result of social pressures rather than any basic biological or psychological differences. Such factors as fear of pregnancy and the double standard by which society has winked at male infidelity, while frowning at the same behavior in women, have tended to create the different patterns. Improved contraception, readily available abortion, and the general liberation of women are acting to remove these restraints on the expression of female sexuality. As a result, infidelity is becoming equally common among both sexes.

The infidelity of either partner is certainly no reason to terminate an otherwise satisfactory marriage. It may, however, be taken as evidence that the needs of the unfaithful partner are not being adequately met within the marriage. If the marriage partners can calmly and rationally discuss their needs and feelings, then the resulting mutual understanding can often result in each partner's being better able to satisfy the needs of the other, so the need for infidelity ceases to exist. A realignment of unrealistic expectations for marriage is often necessary. If a couple cannot work out their own problems, they should not hesitate to seek the help of a qualified marriage counselor. If both partners are willing to "forgive and forget" and work to correct their shortcomings, then even a very shaky marriage may be returned to a state of relative happiness.

Divorce

In some marriages, it becomes apparent that unresolved conflicts have destroyed any basis for continuing the relationship. Marriage can be broken either formally or informally. It may be broken informally by desertion, in which one partner simply disappears, or by separation, in which the couple agree to live separately. Neither desertion nor separation constitutes a legal divorce or terminates the marriage. A marriage can be legally terminated by annulment if it can be established that some legal requirement for marriage was never met (because of fraud, deception, illegal age, bigamy, or some other violation). Or divorce can be obtained if it can be established that one partner violated the marriage rights of the other partner. Technically, in most states, divorce must be based on such grounds rather than on simple mutual agreement. Other states, such as California, have introduced reformed no-fault divorce laws, under which the couple need no grounds other than irreconcilable differences.

Grounds for divorce among the various states include irreconcilable differences, adultery, cruelty (physical or mental), desertion, nonsupport, alcoholism, drug addiction, impotence, insanity, pregnancy at time of marriage, bigamy, fraud, force or duress, felony conviction, and imprisonment. A particular state might recognize many or few of these grounds. Persons seeking divorce often go to extremes to establish complaints within these categories, even though the actual cause of failure was something entirely different. This practice is so common that the number of decrees awarded in certain categories tells very little of the true nature of the marital conflicts among the couples involved.

Incidence of Divorce

The divorce rate in the United States, as shown in Figure 8.1, is at its all-time high. The trend in recent years has been a gradual rise in the divorce rate. Between 1957 and 1974, the rate climbed from 2.2 to about 4.3. The current divorce rate represents 1 divorce for every 2.5 marriages, and it will probably continue to increase in response to more liberal attitudes toward divorce and the reform of laws in many states.

The incidence of divorce can be correlated with several characteristics of the marriage. Divorce occurs more frequently in cities than in rural areas and more often among people of lower income than those of higher income. It is more common during the first five years of marriage than later. Marriages in which one or both parties were less than age 20 at the time of marriage are more likely to end in divorce.

It must be remembered that divorce rates are only a partial indication of marriage failure. Many couples whose marriages have failed have not obtained a divorce for economic or religious reasons, fear of loss of social or professional standing, the presence of children in the home, or fear of admitting failure. The increase in divorce rates is due to many factors, which may or may not include increased unhappiness in marriages. The evolving criteria for success in marriage place a greater importance on love and companionship, without which a marriage today is more often considered to be a failure. Public opinion and divorce laws are increasingly liberal. More and more people are deciding that the temporary pain of

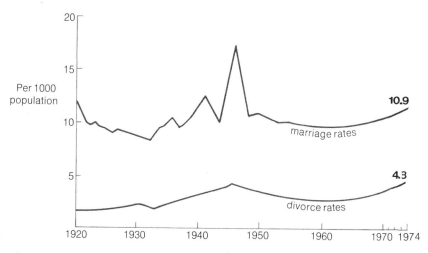

Figure 8.1 *Marriage and divorce rates in the United States, 1920 through 1974.*

divorce is better than living in the continued turmoil of an unhappy marriage. The increasing independence and freedom of women to be self-supporting has probably been influential also.

Remarriage

The remarriage rate among divorcees is high, indicating that few of them are completely soured on the idea of marriage. According to the U.S. Bureau of the Census, a divorced man or woman of any age is more likely to remarry than the never-married person of the same age is to get married initially. The bureau reports, for example, that at age 30 a single woman has a 50 percent chance of marrying, while a divorcee of that age has a 94 percent chance of remarriage.

The divorce rate among second marriages is somewhat higher than in first marriages, while the divorce rate soars in third and subsequent marriages. On the other hand, a remarriage often results in much greater happiness than the original marriage. Remarriages can turn out well if the new partners earnestly try to avoid the problems that destroyed the first marriage.

Summary

I. Individual Readiness for Marriage

    A. Age—chance of success increases with age

    B. Emotional maturity

    C. Social maturity and experience

    D. Financial resources

II. Selecting for Happiness

    A. Positive personality traits—most important

    B. Mutual need satisfaction—good marriage satisfies needs of both partners

    C. Genuine mutual love

    D. Agreement on parenthood

    E. Hereditary traits

    F. Similarity in background:

        1. Age

        2. Ethnic differences

        3. Economic status

        4. Education

        5. Intelligence

6. Religion

G. Danger signals in a relationship—predict problems if marriage should follow:

    1. Quarreling

    2. Lack of communication

    3. Lack of confidence that the marriage will be good

    4. Off-again, on-again relationships

III. Premarital Counseling—can prevent many marital problems

IV. Marital Sexual Adjustment

    A. A sexually inexperienced couple may have anxieties about sexual performance

    B. Should not expect first sexual experiences to be entirely satisfactory

    C. Sexually inexperienced bride may not achieve orgasms for days, weeks, or even months

    D. Open communication of sexual feelings is important

    E. Success of a marriage cannot be measured in terms of orgasms per month

V. Extramarital Sexual Relations

    A. Occur at some time in over half of all marriages

    B. Difficult to pinpoint real causes:

        1. Many people rationalize about their reasons

        2. Causes often nonsexual

    C. May or may not produce guilt

    D Three principal causes:

        1. Lack of commitment

        2. Failure in adjustment

        3. Personality disorders

    E. Old double standard is giving way

    F. Infidelity of either partner no reason to terminate otherwise satisfactory marriage

        1. Should be seen as symptom of problem to be discussed

        2. Marriage counselor may help work out problem

VI. Divorce

    A. Grounds vary among states

B. Incidence

   1. High and rising

   2. Currently 1 divorce for every 2.5 marriages

   3. Rise does not necessarily indicate greater marital unhappiness; may reflect decreasing willingness to tolerate unhappy marriage

C. Many unhappy couples fail to divorce for social, economic, religious, or psychological reasons

D. Remarriage

   1. Rate among divorcees is high

   2. Often results in greater happiness than the original marriage

Questions for Review

1. How do you know whether you are ready for marriage?

2. In nonromantic terms, what is a good marriage?

3. What traits should you look for in a potential marriage partner?

4. What traits do you look for?

5. Which of your needs would you expect a good marriage to fulfill?

6. What patterns in a relationship portend problems if the couple should marry?

7. How can a couple achieve a satisfactory sexual adjustment?

8. Why do married people enter into extramarital involvements?

9. How should a couple handle the situation of infidelity on the part of one or both?

10. Why do you think the divorce rate is so rapidly rising?

GLOSSARY

abortion | Premature expulsion from the uterus of the product of conception—the embryo or nonviable fetus.

afterbirth | The placenta and other membranes cast from the uterus after the birth of the child.

age of consent | The minimum age by law for a person to consent legally to sexual intercourse.

amniocentesis | Withdrawal of a sample of amniotic fluid for detection of fetal defects or determination of fetal sex.

amnion | Membrane that surrounds the embryo within the uterus, secreting amniotic fluid to form the "bag of waters."

amniotic fluid | Fluid produced by the amnion early in pregnancy.

ampulla | Dilated secton of a tubular structure.

androgen | A masculinizing hormone.

annulment | The legal dissolving of a marital relationship on grounds the marriage was not valid according to the laws of the state.

anterior pituitary gland | The front, or anterior, lobe of the pituitary gland, which is located at the base of the brain.

artificial insemination	Introduction of semen into the uterus by artificial means.
bestiality	Engaging in sexual contact with animals.
bisexuality	Feeling sexual attraction for both males and females.
bulbourethral glands	Pair of small glands located in the lower abdomen of the male, secreting a lubricating fluid into the urethra upon sexual arousal and contributing a small amount of fluid to the semen.
castration	Removal of the gonads.
cervix	The lower, narrow, necklike portion of the uterus.
cesarean section	Incision through the abdominal and uterine walls for delivery of a fetus; done when birth through the natural passages is impossible or dangerous.
chorion	Outermost embryonic membrane, part of which unites with the uterine lining to form the placenta.
chorionic gonadotropin	The gonadotropic substance from human placentas.
chorionic villi	Threadlike projections growing in tufts on the external surface of the chorion; a part of the fetal portion of the placenta.
chromosome	Small, rod-shaped body which appears in the nucleus of a cell at the time of cell division; carries the genes.
cilia	Minute, hairlike structures capable of a waving motion and attached to the outer surface of cells; responsible for movement of the ovum through the fallopian tube.
circumcision	Removal of all or a part of the foreskin of the penis.
climacteric	Pertaining to the various physical and mental changes occurring at the termination of the reproductive years in the female.
clitoris	Small, erectile sensory structure located at forward juncture of the vulva of female external genitals.
coitus	Sexual intercourse.

colostrum	Thin, milky fluid secreted by the mammary gland a few days both before and after delivery.
common-law marriage	An agreement between a man and a woman to enter into a marriage relationship without either a church or civil ceremony; not recognized as legal in most states.
conception	Fertilization of the ovum to produce an embryo.
condom	Sheath or cover for the penis, worn during intercourse to prevent impregnation and/or disease.
contraception	The prevention of pregnancy.
contraceptive	A device for the prevention of pregnancy.
corpora cavernosa	Two columns of erectile tissue on either side of the penis.
corpus luteum	Ovarian follicle after discharge of the ovum, persisting as a yellow mass that secretes ovarian hormones.
corpus spongiosum	Column of erectile tissue that forms the urethral surface of the penis.
cunnilingus	Oral stimulation of the clitoris, labia, and vagina.
decidua	Tissue of the uterine lining surrounding the embryo following the time of implantation.
desertion	The act of abandoning a marriage partner.
diaphragm	Rubber or plastic device fitted over the cervix to prevent entrance of sperm into the uterus.
divorce	The legal dissolving of a marriage.
donor insemination	Artificial insemination in which the semen used is that of a man other than the woman's husband.
douche	Irrigation of the vaginal cavity with water or spermicide to kill and wash out sperm.
Down's syndrome	Mongolism.
ejaculation	Expulsion of the semen during male orgasm.
ejaculatory duct	Duct carrying semen form the seminal vesicle to the prostate gland.

embryo	Early developing stage of any organism; in the human, refers to developing organism during the first eight weeks.
endocrine glands	Glands that secrete into the blood a substance (hormone) that acts elsewhere in the body.
endometrium	Mucous membrane lining the inside of the uterus.
epididymis	Oblong body attached to each testis, in which sperm cells mature and are stored.
erection	The condition in which the penis becomes rigid and elevated.
erythroblastosis fetalis	An anemia of the fetus or newborn infant arising from a blood incompatibility (usually Rh) between the fetus and the mother.
estrogen	Female sex hormone, promoting female sexual development.
exhibitionism	In general, the display of sex organs for the purpose of attracting sexual interest; more specifically, the exposure of the penis to an unsuspecting female as a final sexual gratification without any intention of further sexual contact.
extrauterine	Situated or occurring outside the uterus.
eunuch	A male deprived of the testes before puberty.
fallopian tubes	Pair of ducts carrying the ova from the ovaries to the uterus; also called oviducts.
fellatio	Oral stimulation or manipulation of the penis.
fertilization	Fusion of a sperm with an ovum, creating the zygote.
fetishism	Sexual arousal from the perception of inanimate objects; the worship of an inanimate object as a symbol of a loved person.
fetus	Unborn child after eight weeks of development.
follicle-stimulating hormone (FSH)	Gonadotropic hormone from the anterior pituitary gland, stimulating the maturation of the ovarian follicle and its production of estrogens.

foreskin	Covering fold of skin over the glans penis; also called the prepuce.
fraternal twins	Twins who have developed from two different zygotes, or fertilized eggs; nonidentical.
genitalia	The reproductive organs. The external genitalia are those on the outside of the body.
glans penis	Cap-shaped expansion of the corpus spongiosum at the end of the penis.
gonad	An ovary or testis.
gonadotropic hormone	Any gonad-stimulating hormone.
graafian follicle	Maturing ovarian follicle, containing the ovum.
heterosexuality	Feeling sexual attraction for persons of the opposite sex.
homosexuality	Feeling sexual attraction for persons of the same sex.
hormone	A chemical substance produced by one organ and carried by the blood to exert a specific effect on another organ.
hymen	The membranous fold that partially closes the external opening of the vagina.
hysterectomy	Surgical removal of the uterus.
identical twins	Twins who have developed from a single zygote, or fertilized egg.
implantation	Attachment of the embryo to the lining of the uterus and its subsequent penetration of and embedding in that lining.
impotence	Incapacity for sexual intercourse in the male; may be physical or emotional in origin.
incest	Sexual intercourse between individuals too closely related to marry legally.
induced abortion	Abortion produced artificially.

infertility   Temporary inability to conceive or to induce conception.

interstitial cell   Cell lying between the seminiferous tubules of the testes, secreting testosterone.

intrauterine device   Device placed within the uterus to prevent conception
(IUD)   or implantation.

labia   Liplike portions of the female external genitals.

labia majora   The outer, larger, liplike portions of the female external genitals.

labia minora   The inner, smaller, liplike portions of the female external genitals.

labor   The series of processes by which the baby and other products of conception are expelled from the body of the mother.

lactation   The secretion of milk.

lesbianism   Homosexuality between females.

luteinizing hormone   Hormone from the anterior pituitary which stimulates
(LH)   corpus luteum formation in the ovary and the secretion of testosterone by the testis.

luteotropic hormone   Hormone from the anterior pituitary that stimulates
(LTH)   progesterone secretion by the corpus luteum and causes the breasts to produce milk.

masochism   Attainment of sexual satisfaction from suffering physical pain.

masturbation   Production of orgasm by self-manipulation of the sex organs.

menarche   Beginning of the menstrual cycle in adolescence.

menopause   Cessation of menstruation, occurring usually between ages 45 and 50.

menstrual cycle   Regularly recurring cycle of physiological events, including ovulation and menstruation.

menstruation   Cyclic uterine bleeding resulting from degeneration of the lining of the uterus.

miscarriage	A natural, or spontaneous, abortion.
mongolism	A condition resulting from the presence of one extra chromosome or piece of chromosome in each body cell; Down's syndrome.
mons veneris	Rounded fleshy prominence over the pubis of the female.
nocturnal emission	Discharge of semen (seminal fluid) during sleep; commonly begins shortly after puberty.
nucleus	Spheroid body within a cell, containing the chromosomes.
orgasm	Climax of sexual excitement.
ovarian follicle	The egg and its encasing cells at any stage of its development.
ovary	Female gonad, in which ova and hormones are formed.
oviduct	Fallopian tube, carrying ova from the ovary to the uterus.
ovulation	Discharge of the mature egg from the Graafian follicle of the ovary.
ovum	Egg (sex cell).
pedophilia	Sexual involvement of an adult with a child.
penis	Male organ of copulation
pituitary gland	Gland located at the base of the brain; secretes numerous hormones, many of which stimulate the function of the other hormone-producing glands; also called the hypophysis.
placenta	Disc-shaped organ formed within the uterus during pregnancy through which materials are exchanged between maternal and fetal blood.
presentation	First part of the child to make its appearance in delivery.
progesterone	Hormone produced by the corpus luteum, promoting the maturity of the uterine lining and its maintenance during pregnancy.

progestin	Synthetic progesterone.
prostate gland	Gland in the male surrounding the neck of the bladder and the urethra.
puberty	Period of time during which sexual maturity is achieved.
Rh factor	A chemical substance present in red blood cells of most people. Those possessing it are Rh+, those lacking it are Rh−
sadism	Attainment of sexual satisfaction from the infliction of pain on another person.
scrotum	Sac that contains the testes and related structures.
secondary sex characteristics	Characteristics specific to the male or female but not directly concerned with reproduction.
semen	Product of the male reproductive organs, a mixture of spermatozoa and fluid secretions from the prostate and various other glands and cells.
seminal vesicle	Gland located on each vas deferens; the primary source of the fluid portion of the semen.
seminiferous tubules	Numerous small tubes in the testis; the site of sperm production.
sperm	Mature male germ cell; sperm cell, spermatozoon.
spermicide	Any agent that destroys spermatozoa.
sterility	Total inability to produce offspring.
suppository	Medicated mass to be introduced into an orifice of the body.
term	Culmination of pregnancy at the end of ten lunar months or slightly over nine calendar months.
testis	Male gonad, producing spermatozoa and testosterone.
testosterone	Male sex hormone, produced by the testes, inducing male secondary sex characteristics.

toxemias	A group of conditions occurring in pregnant women, including high blood pressure, excess fluid in the tissues, and albumin in the urine.
transvestism	Wearing the clothing of the opposite sex for the emotional or sexual gratification it provides.
trimester	One-third of the term of pregnancy, or thirteen weeks.
tubal ligation	Surgical procedure to tie off the oviducts.
umbilical cord	Flexible structure connecting the umbilicus with the placenta and giving passage to the umbilical arteries and veins.
urethra	Duct carrying urine from the bladder to the exterior of the body; also carries semen in the male.
uterus	Hollow, muscular, pear-shaped organ of the female in which the fetus develops.
vagina	The sheathlike structure in the female that receives the penis in intercourse; also the birth canal.
vas deferens	Duct carrying sperm from the testis to the seminal vesicles.
vasectomy	Surgical removal of a portion of the vas deferens.
voyeurism	Attainment of sexual gratification by looking at sexual objects or situations.
vulva	External genital organs of the female.
zygote	Cell resulting from the fusion of the sperm and egg; the fertilized ovum.

BIBLIOGRAPHY

Aaron, Ruth. "Male Contributions to Female Frigidity." *Medical Aspects of Human Sexuality* 5, no. 5 (May 1971): 42–57.

Auerback, Alfred. "Nymphomania." *Medical Aspects of Human Sexuality* 6, no. 6 (June 1972): 9.

Bardwick, Judith. *Psychology of Women.* New York: Harper & Row, 1971.

Bauman, Karl E. "Selected Aspects of the Contraceptive Practices of Unmarried University Students." *Medical Aspects of Human Sexuality* 5, no. 8 (August 1971): 76–89.

Connell, Elizabeth B. "The IUD: Sex Without Pregnancy." *Medical Aspects of Human Sexuality* 6, no. 1 (January 1972): 142–167.

Crawshaw, Ralph. "The Psychology of the Unwed Mother." *Medical Aspects of Human Sexuality* 5, no. 6 (June 1971): 176–188.

Debrovner, Charles H. "Sexual and Medical Considerations of Contraception." *Medical Aspects of Human Sexuality* 5, no. 10 (October 1971): 118–151.

Gebhard, Paul, et al. *Sex Offenders.* New York: Harper & Row, 1965.

Grant, Igor. "Anxiety About Orgasm." *Medical Aspects of Human Sexuality* 6, no. 3 (March 1972): 14–46.

Guyton, Arthur C. *Textbook of Medical Physiology.* 4th ed. Philadelphia: Saunders, 1971.

Hayman, Charles, and Lanza, Charlene. "Victimology of Sexual Assault." *Medical Aspects of Human Sexuality* 5, no. 10 (October 1971): 152–161.

Hellman, Louis M., and Pritchard, Jack A. Williams. *Obstetrics.* 14th ed. New York: Appleton, 1971.

"Infertility." *Medical World News* 10, no. 40 (9 October 1970): 32–39.

Jones, Kenneth L., Shainberg, Louis W., and Byer, Curtis O. *Health Science.* 3rd ed. New York: Harper & Row, 1974.

Kaplan, Helen A., and Sager, Clifford J. "Sexual Response at Different Ages." *Medical Aspects of Human Sexuality* 5, no. 6 (June 1971): 10–23.

Katz, Jack. "Biological and Psychological Roots of Psychosexual Identity." *Medical Aspects of Human Sexuality* 6, no. 6 (June 1972): 102–116.

Kinsey, Alfred C., et al. *Sexual Behavior in the Human Female.* Philadelphia: Saunders, 1953.

Kinsey, Alfred C., et al. *Sexual Behavior in the Human Male.* Philadelphia: Saunders, 1948.

Kozol, Harry. "Myths About the Sexual Offender." *Medical Aspects of Human Sexuality* 5, no. 6 (June 1971): 50–65.

Lehfeldt, Hans. "Psychology of Contraceptive Failure." *Medical Aspects of Human Sexuality* 5, no. 5 (May 1971): 68–79.

Masters, William H., and Johnson, Virginia E. *Human Sexual Inadequacy.* Boston: Little, Brown, 1970.

Masters, William H., and Johnson, Virginia E. *Human Sexual Response.* Boston: Little, Brown, 1966.

Masters, William H., and Johnson, Virginia E. "A Pictorial Review of the Stages of Sexual Response in Women." *Medical Aspects of Human Sexuality* 4, no. 7 (July 1970): 9–20.

Mohr, J.W., Turner, R. E. and Jerry, M. B. *Pedophilia and Exhibitionism.* Toronto: University of Toronto Press, 1964.

Ovesey, Lionel, and Meyers, Helen. "Retarded Ejaculation." *Medical Aspects of Human Sexuality* 4, no. 11 (November 1970): 98–119.

Peters, Joseph, and Sadoff, Robert. "Clinical Observations on Child Molesters." *Medical Aspects of Human Sexuality* 4, no. 11 (November 1970): 20–33.

Racy, John. "Ten Misuses of Sex." *Medical Aspects of Human Sexuality* 5, no. 2 (February 1971): 136–145.

Remarriages, United States. U.S. Department of Health, Education, and Welfare Publication No. (HRA) 74-1903, December 1973.

Roth, Russell. "The Brave New World of the Transsexuals." *Modern Medicine* (21 February 1972): 156–161.

Salzman, Leon. "Female Infidelity." *Medical Aspects of Human Sexuality* 6, no. 2 (February 1972): 118–136.

Salzman, Leon. "Premature Ejaculation." *Medical Aspects of Human Sexuality* 6, no. 6 (June 1972): 118–127.

Soloman, Philip, and Patch, Vernon. *Handbook of Psychiatry.* 2nd ed. Los Altos, Calif.: Lange Medical Publications, 1971.

Stanley, Elizabeth. "Female Sexual Arousal." *Medical Aspects of Human Sexuality* 8, no. 2 (February 1974): 98-133.

Ziegal, Erna, and Van Blarcom, Carolyn. *Obstetric Nursing.* 6th ed. New York: Macmillan, 1972.

Zinsser, Hans H. "Surgical Sterilization." *Medical Aspects of Human Sexuality* 5, no. 8 (August 1971): 102–109.

INDEX

Numbers in italics refer to pages containing tables or figures.